SEARCHING TO BE FOUND

SEARCHING TO BE FOUND

Understanding and Helping Adopted and Looked After Children with Attention Difficulties

Randy Lee Comfort

Routledge
Taylor & Francis Group
LONDON AND NEW YORK

First published 2008 by
Karnac Books Ltd.

Published 2022 by Routledge
2 Park Square, Milton Park, Abingdon, Oxon OX14 4RN
605 Third Avenue, New York, NY 10017

Routledge is an imprint of the Taylor & Francis Group, an informa business

First issued in hardback 2019

British Library Cataloguing in Publication Data

A C.I.P. for this book is available from the British Library

ISBN-13: 978-1-85575-464-5 (pbk)
ISBN-13: 978-0-367-32674-6 (hbk)

Edited, designed and produced by The Studio Publishing Services Ltd
www.publishingservicesuk.co.uk
e-mail: studio@publishingservicesuk.co.uk

CONTENTS

This book is dedicated to the families of Our Place

ACKNOWLEDGEMENTS

I am deeply grateful to the Trustees, the staff, the families, and the children at Our Place who have put the meat on the bones of my research and my professional thinking. Each of you has taught me so much more than any one of you realizes.

I am indebted to my friend and colleague, Margaret Borkowski, whose eagle eye and keen sensitivity have contributed enormously to my writing. I would also like to thank Susan Pizzolato for making such astute comments on the initial manuscript.

My four children are foremost in everything I do, and they are an integral part of all that I have learned and shared with others. My gratitude is always for them and to them.

ABOUT THE AUTHOR

Randy Lee Comfort graduated from Smith College in Massachusetts and received a Master's Degree in Social Work from the University of Pennsylvania, followed by a Doctorate in Educational Psychology from the University of Denver. She has worked for over thirty-five years in the fields of family counselling, learning disorders, and adoption and fostering. Dr Comfort is the mother of both biological and adopted children.

After living, working, and bringing up her children in the USA, Dr Comfort moved to Bristol, in the UK, where, in 1998, she opened Our Place: a Centre for Families who Foster and Adopt. In addition to running Our Place, she continues to lecture internationally on the topics of learning disorders and adoption/fostering, and pursues her career in writing about and counselling these children and their families.

Dr Comfort is the author of *The Unconventional Child; Teaching the Unconventional Child; The Child Care Catalog*; numerous journal articles; and chapters in edited books. Since the late 1980s, she has taught teachers and social workers about attention deficit disorders, adoption/fostering issues, and social dysfunctions as a part of her teaching in special needs education classes.

PREFACE

Working with families who foster and adopt, as well as with children having various learning and living difficulties, I am frequently meeting with adoptive parents, foster carers, social workers and teachers who ask if I think the child we are discussing has an attention deficit hyperactivity disorder. This is a question I am reluctant to answer directly or specifically because large numbers of children who are, or have been, in the care system present with characteristics that are similar, sometimes almost identical, to the symptoms of an attention deficit disorder. Difficulties with concentration, focus and attentiveness are extremely common in the looked after and adopted population. Moreover, many of these children also behave unpredictably, aggressively, and erratically. On normative checklists, children with an attention deficit hyperactivity disorder (ADHD) or an attention deficit disorder (ADD) and adopted/looked after children can achieve the same scores and comments.

The dilemma that arises for me in my hesitancy to respond to the question coincides with the fact that there is no definitive diagnosis for ADHD/ADD. I need to wonder if the child's behaviour is a reflection of traumatic early life events or if the child, under optimal circumstances, would have acted in this manner anyway. In both situations, there will be neurological dysfunctions and chemical imbalances undermining the brain's ability to manage effectively. The intervention and treatment, which frequently can be the same or similar regardless of the origin of the dysfunction, sometimes does need to differ. Not categorically, not always, but usually, it is my professional view that issues surrounding adoption/fostering need to take precedence over concerns about ADHD/ADD if, at any specific time, one has to choose.

Although "adoption" and "being in care" are definable terms, ADHD/ADD is not. Nevertheless, within a playing field that has rough parameters, if not staked goal posts, professionals have all developed their own versions of what the criteria for an attention disorder entails. Equally, each of us continuously applies our own theoretical knowledge, individual bias, personal experience and subjective judgment to interpreting the data that result from a child's assessment and evaluation. In doing so, we organise our own psychological thinking about how to work with a child, a family, schools and communities. In some situations, this is easier or clearer to do than in others, but both adoption/being in care and ADHD/ADD make evaluation and therapeutic intervention very complicated.

The concern in this book is not one of a diagnosis of ADHD/ADD, although it certainly is highly recommended that a child presenting with attention disorders has access to a thorough developmental assessment. Rather, the book is an attempt to provide a comprehensive perspective on adopted/looked after children who cause problems for themselves and others because of their attention disorders and concomitant behavioural difficulties, and to suggest meaningful and practical strategies that can lead to improvement in the short term as well as long term for the children, their families, their teachers and others in their social circles.

In the twenty-first century, virtually everyone concurs that the interplay between genetics and the environment is crucial to a child's development. Almost daily, there is new and exciting research in the fields of neurobiology and neuropsychology that enhances our understanding of how the brain develops and what the effects of both nature and nurture can have on the developing child. The insights provided by this research often require that we reconsider how we conceptualise and work with children who have been exposed to extended periods of trauma and children who display a variety of developmental weaknesses. Knowing that adopted/looked after children as well as children with attentional difficulties have experienced dysfunction in their lives, it is useful to think, not only about the theoretical causes and consequences, but also about the practical implications for intervention and treatment with affected children.

Searching to Be Found addresses the association between children who are adopted or looked after and who manifest significant difficulties with attention and the behaviours most usually associated with an attention deficit disorder. As the aim of the book is to better understand and treat the behaviours, emotions and needs of adopted/looked after children with attention problems, no single approach to behaviour management has been advocated, no particular theoretical model has been endorsed, and there has been no attempt to discuss the pros and cons of medication. The intent has consistently been to understand where the child is coming from, to think about what an individual child might be needing, and to consider the most efficacious means of providing an environment in which the child has a better chance to grow and develop. Diet, exercise, medication, a change of school, a friend, a new leisure activity, a sensitive therapist, a book or a piece of music can each and all be possible factors of an equation that may produce a better functioning and happier child, and thereby the family and teacher as well.

Since many have asked, the title of this book derives from my personal interpretations of the stories children and their families tell me. Alone and desperate, children in the care system are constantly looking for ways to allow someone to find them - not just find them a home or a family, but to help them define and discover who they really are. Children with attention dysfunctions are equally lost, and are therefore just as needy of being found. All of these children do everything they possibly can, positively or negatively, to access the attention they require in order to get along in the world in which they live. Fight as they might, each child is determined to find the caring adult or friend who will walk through the forest with him/her so that they can come out together on the other side. Whether adopted, looked after, ADHD, ADD or any combination of these, all of these children are expectantly and hopefully searching to be found.

The focus of this book, therefore, is to provide children, parents, carers and professionals with a few maps with which to negotiate the forest. Fortuitously, there is not a single road to travel, but a variety of paths to try and to follow. Some will work better than others depending upon a host of factors influencing the particular child and his or her circumstances. Some will walk faster than others, and many will have to retrace quite a few steps, but it is to be remembered that the only way out is through.

The first chapter of the book helps to define who are children in care and what their backgrounds and being in care may mean to them. The secret stories and the inescapable black plastic bag travel of their early years are opened for inspection with the intent of helping parents, carers and teachers to better understand the shadows that do not fall behind when the sun sets.

The second chapter seeks to describe in accessible terminology how the infant brain grows and what it needs for this process. The role of both heredity and the environment on neurodevelopment is seen to be critical in influencing the child's course of overall development, although, inexplicably and most wonderously, there are always children who defy the odds. Moreover, there is scientifically based research indicating that the plasticity of the brain allows for healing, improvement, resilience, and progress.

The next two chapters address very specific strategies for living with and teaching the ADHD/ADD adopted/looked after child at home, in the community and in school. It is consistently stressed throughout this book that magic, recipes, easy answers and one-size-fits-all approaches are antithetical to the philosophy of how and why I like to work with unconventional children. These chapters offer a multitude of ideas and creative interventions that have been designed as examples to inspire parents, carers, teachers, social workers and therapists to try to know and understand the specific child and to establish a programme with and for that child which has a good chance of being successful because it is so personally individualised.

Chapter Five explores the social development of the ADHD/ADD adopted and looked after child, again seeking ways and means of enhancing a child's self esteem and self confidence by recognising what activities, interests, friends and outlets specifically suit the child in question. In this chapter, the reader will also be referred to a variety of specific games and books that may be useful when living/working with children who suffer from low self image.

One of the biggest difficulties in writing a book of this nature is the ever-changing field of knowledge that is developing so rapidly. Each time I thought I had completed a chapter, I read something new, or heard a child differently, or listened to insightful feedback from a parent/carer that necessitated a reconsideration of what I had just written. This is exciting. It is also frustrating because one closes with a sense of not being quite finished. On the other hand, I haven't wanted the book to be an ending; my hope is that it will mark the beginning for parents, carers, teachers and other professionals to reconsider their own approaches to living with and learning from adopted/looked after children who have attention disorders.

CHAPTER ONE

The adopted/looked after child with attention difficulties

Daniel squirms in the chair, his small legs already running, while his large, sparkling eyes watch the tears dripping into Shirley's lap. He sees the wet stain growing wider on his new mother's summer skirt, and waits impatiently for her to talk, but she doesn't say a word. Before he can stop himself, Daniel moves impulsively toward the playroom door, knocking over the paint jar and splattering the brushes to the floor.

"Are all adopted children like this?" Shirley asks the therapist.

Meanwhile, Daniel's older sister, Christie, who is in long-term foster care, is a quiet, distant, inattentive child. Her carers question her suitability for adoption because she is so withdrawn and aloof.

"How can we brighten up this little girl?" they ask their therapist.

According to informal reporting, it would seem that a disproportionate number of foster carers and adopters live with children who manifest attention difficulties, usually, but not always, with hyperactivity. While it is clear that adoption or being in care does not cause a child to have Attention Deficit Hyperactivity Disorder/Attention Deficit Disorder (ADHD/ADD), and while having ADHD / ADD does not determine whether or not a child will be taken into care, the association between children who are or have been in the care system and those with attention difficulties is frequently discussed. This relationship, whether clinically proven or just anecdote-based is an important one to understand as parents, carers, teachers, and professionals struggle to meet the needs of a group of children who are at high risk for academic and social failure. Both ADHD / ADD and adopted / looked after children who do not receive the creative intervention they require contribute to the tragic statistics currently describing these groups of children—young people who are vulnerable to loneliness, homelessness, academic underachievement, difficulty getting along with peers, problems dealing with authority, use and abuse of substances, high rates of teen pregnancy, under-employment, and repetitive prison sentences.

Sensitive and multi-modal frameworks for thinking about each child individually are especially useful when living and working with the adopted / looked after child who brings a disruptive early childhood experience into the family and the school. Often, these disturbing and dysfunctional backgrounds help to explain the child's inattentive and impulsive behaviour. It is equally important to provide a holistic framework for the child whose neurobiological make-up leads him to be aggressive, hostile, disorganized, and unregulated—factors that may or may not have contributed to his / her coming into the care system.

Broadly speaking, ADHD / ADD is usually viewed as a developmental disorder of self-control that consists of problems with attention span, impulse control, and activity level that lead to impairment of the child's ability to function successfully at home and at school. Some children display these characteristics without being hyperactive as well, and are referred to as children with ADD rather than ADHD. Both of these conditions are characterized by symptoms of inattention, impulsivity, distractibility, and erratic levels of performance. Since this disorder is defined behaviourally (there is no definitive diagnosis for ADHD / ADD), it is inevitable that some children with other neurological, psychosocial or learning disorders may appear to meet some or all of the criteria established for a diagnosis of ADHD / ADD (Nigg, 2006). Children who have been traumatized by violence, abuse, exposure to drugs, neglect, and separation from the birth parent could meet many or most of the ADHD/ADD criteria. (See Appendix I)

Adopted children are those who live with a permanent family other than their birth parents. Virtually all adopted children have been living outside their birth family prior to being adopted. The length of time they live in foster care varies enormously. Looked after children are those who are in some form of temporary care, usually in a foster home, although possibly in a group home. Whether deemed "short-term" or "long-term" care, many of these placements are not enduring, resulting in frequent moves for the looked after child. An increasing number of looked after children are living with relatives in what is now referred to as "kinship care".

It is not the intention of this book to determine whether or not a child has a clinical attention deficit, but to accept the fact that there are many adopted/looked after children whose lives, which are already complicated and often traumatized, are made even more difficult by their attention dysfunctions. As such, a better understanding of how both neurobiological and psycho-emotional experiences have equipped the ADHD/ADD adopted/looked after child to think and behave will form the basis for considering how to formulate creative and child-specific strategies for improving the child's overall well-being.

Many adopters and foster carers speak frequently and frantically about the inexplicable behaviours of children who come into their homes. Often their concerns focus on the behavioural difficulties, aggression, hyperactivity, and inattention of the children in their care. Shirley is far from alone when she asks her therapist if "all adopted children are like this?" As social workers often do not have full information on a child's background, and since most foster carers and adoptive parents receive little or no specific training and education about how to live with and manage children who have been abused and traumatized, they can be overwhelmed by behaviours that are so wide of the mark from anything they have experienced before with other children. Moreover, the particular needs of a child with an attention disorder can be extremely perplexing and exhausting to parents or carers who are trying to put into place all of the love and affection and positive discipline that have worked for them before.

The paucity of literature addressing ADHD/ADD adopted/looked after children and their families and teachers may reflect the difficulty one encounters in trying to understand (1) the complexity of environmental and psycho-social factors that any given child brings into a new family; and (2) the fact that it is so hard for the medical and psychological professions to agree upon a definition of ADHD. Nevertheless, those who live and work with these children recognize the need for help and intervention—both for the child and for the adults responsible for the child's care and learning.

The persistent questions asked by carers, adoptive parents and professionals include:

- Why is ADHD/ADD so prevalent in the care system?
- Is ADHD/ADD a cause or effect of adoption/being looked after?
- Is being in care/adopted a cause or effect of attention difficulties?
- Are adopted/looked after children really more likely to suffer from ADHD/ADD than are children who are not or have not been in the care system, or is that a myth?

Clearly, there are no simple or straightforward answers to these questions, although it is important to address the issues arising from these concerns, which is what this book proposes to do.

The issue of ADHD/ADD itself is complex, and there is considerable professional controversy about what ADHD/ADD is and is not. Among the questions these professionals debate are the issues of what it actually is and how it can be defined (medically and socially):

- does ADHD/ADD even exist as a proper diagnosis or condition?
- is it a neurological deficit?
- is it the result of poor behaviour management or negligent upbringing?

Since the professionals are still struggling with how to define, diagnose, and treat attention deficits, it is no wonder that parents, carers, and teachers are confused about how to handle the ADHD/

ADD child. The situation becomes that much more duplicitous and worrisome if the ADHD/ADD child is also adopted or in care. Teachers, usually more so than parents and carers, can vary widely in their approach to such children.

> Mrs Belgrade is not familiar with ADHD. It is her view that teachers teach children and all children are different anyway. Her premise is that she has a certain amount of material to teach in Year 3, and that is what she will teach. Mrs Belgrade makes an effort to engage the children and to teach in a variety of modalities, but that is as far as she will go.
>
> Mr Tuner thinks that he probably has an attention deficit himself, and he quickly gets bored teaching the National Curriculum; therefore, he presents material in the most intriguing ways he can think of, and hopes it comes through to at least several children on any given day. Mr Tuner worries a lot about the children in the care system, as he had considerable experience teaching them previously, so he goes out of his way to make accommodations for these children and their families.
>
> Ms Frances is in her first year of teaching and is totally overwhelmed by her class of thirty students, two of whom she knows are adopted and one of whom she expects has ADHD. She has been taught to think about early childhood development and she knows that many children come to school with various learning disorders, but nothing has prepared her for the activity and emotional level that the adopted/ADHD child has presented from day one. She wants to help and to individualize her curriculum for this student, but has no idea how and what to do.

When it is thought that a child might fall into the spectrum of an attention disorder, it is extremely important that a multi-diagnostic team contribute to the child's evaluation because there is no biological, neurological or physiological test that can confirm such a diagnosis in and of itself. A multi-diagnostic team will want to include:

- documentation of specific attention deficit traits from parents, teachers, and others directly associated with the child;
- a comprehensive physical examination to rule out other medical conditions that may be contributing to or interfering with normal developmental functioning;

- evaluation of other neurodevelopmental dysfunctions that might be associated with attention deficits, such as processing problems, motor or speech and language delays, social and cognitive incongruities;
- a psychological or psychiatric evaluation of the child's mental health that might reveal associated or secondary problem areas: learning disorders, anxiety, depression, trauma, attachment difficulties, etc.;
- a psycho-educational assessment that includes intellectual ability and an evaluation of specific learning disorders and learning styles. An overview of the child's social and behavioural functioning at school as well as the academic standing of the child should be considered;
- a social worker's assessment of the familial situation and home environment.

Although a comprehensive evaluation can be extremely helpful in many ways, nothing is definitive in the area of ADHD/ADD, and, as shall be seen, children who come into the care system often bring with them similar traits to those children who are categorized as ADHD/ADD. Sometimes, the adopted/looked after child may mirror characteristics that are so closely associated with ADHD/ADD that one can hardly tease apart which is which. This also broaches the question of whether an infant's very difficult temperament and behaviour (possible ADHD/ADD), may have contributed to poor parental handling and upbringing, and/or whether this infant's propensity to become an individual with attention problems was exacerbated by the environment in which the child lived prior to entering care. There are babies who are hard to cuddle, to soothe, to engage. If a fragile mother or father is already dealing with compelling personal disruptions, parenting a child of this disposition will not be an easy task.

The recommended treatment for children with ADHD/ADD also varies enormously. Behavioural therapy, involving a system of rewards and consequences, has been the most common approach; however, cognitive behavioural therapy, in which the child is taught to think specifically about his behaviours, is another frequently used form of therapeutic intervention. Some therapists concentrate on helping parents to develop skills for managing and redirecting behaviour that has become out of control. An alternative approach to behaviour management is through diet (cutting out additives and sugars and making various food group adjustments); while yet another, more psychodynamic therapeutic strategy would be that of focusing on a child's past history, helping him to come to terms with his early experiences. Some therapists might be inclined to concentrate on the neurological components and brain development, paying particular attention to early child development. At times, medication is advised, and has proved to be extremely helpful in well managed cases. Currently, more professionals are looking at non-invasive therapeutic procedures that can help to reorganize neural pathways. Physical and occupational therapists have been using these techniques for many years in their work with children suffering from a variety of sensory integration disorders. Most therapists would utilize some of each and all of these approaches, but any given therapist might have a particular inclination to pursue one line of thinking more strongly than another.

* * *

> "Memory was trauma, and memory was all they had, primal memories of a type it is impossible to forget" (Grant, 2006, p. 185).

Both Daniel and Christie are complicated children who reflect the difficulties presented by many children in the care system and who manifest a variety of dysfunctional behaviours. Even the professionals trying to assess and help these children and their families struggle to come to definitive diagnoses and evaluations of children who present with symptoms that can be mistaken for one condition or another. Indeed, it is not unanticipated that many adoptive parents and carers will wonder how much being adopted/looked after enters into the equation of a child's disruptive behaviours and emotions. Most families who take in a child with unruly and unpredictable behaviour, a child who does not sit still and cannot follow through on tasks, a child who acts impulsively and appears to be terribly scattered in all aspects of life, inevitably will question the possibility of an attention disorder.

Since Christie does not display the rambunctious, frenetic behaviour of her brother, she is less likely to be thought of as a child with attention problems. She might be thought to have a low IQ or attachment difficulties. She may be seen as being excessively shy and withdrawn. Children with attention difficulties who do not also have hyperactivity (more frequently girls than boys) are often overlooked or improperly labelled as they do not command the immediate attention of teachers, parents, and care-takers.

> In fact, Christie's foster carer was not considering ADD when she talked to the therapist about Christie. This was a woman who knew very little about Christie's background—in this case, no fault of the social worker's, who also had little or no idea of what Christie had been through—but was trying to help a little girl to become more involved with the world around her. At the same time, Christie was afraid of that world, and was making every effort to withdraw from it; but, this was not known to her carers or social worker, and Christie was unable to express these feelings herself.
>
> Concomitantly, however, Christie's inherited attention deficit disorder made thinking coherently and sequentially about what was going on in her life an even more difficult task.

In an ideal world, both Christie and Daniel would benefit from a comprehensive assessment of their cognitive, educational, medical, emotional, and psycho-social functioning; yet, both are children whose attention disorders are not easily explained, even with very expert evaluation, because their early childhood years were so fraught with traumatic disturbances.

Being adopted or looked after is more concrete than being ADHD/ADD. A child either is or is not adopted/looked after, although children living in "kinship" care situations and those in very short-term care can be somewhat harder to define and describe. Usually, because adoption and fostering are more specific than is ADHD/ADD, less controversy exists among professionals who write about children looked after or adopted than among professionals investigating ADHD/ADD.

In the field of adoption, even nature *vs.* nurture is not much of an issue any more. The question is not *if* the environment can make a difference, but *when* and *how* it can make a difference. Although there is general agreement that genetics play a role, the exact interplay of genes and environment is not clear-cut either.

All researchers working in the adoption/fostering field agree that for most children in the care system in contemporary society, there will have been substantial experience of neglect, possibly malnutrition, feasibly domestic violence, and usually inadequate cognitive and emotional stimulation. Moreover, in many instances, there also will have been physical, sexual, and/or emotional abuse. Frequently, exposure to adults who substance-abuse is also a part of the child's environment. Experts agree that there may be neurological, intellectual, physical, emotional, and social consequences resulting from these injurious situations. At the very least, each and all of these children will have suffered to some degree from separation anxieties.

One can theorize about ADHD/ADD adopted/looked after children for a long time, or one can assume a more practical approach. *Searching to Be Found* has taken a practice-based orientation, which tries to formulate a plan of intervention that is based on research and theoretical knowledge of complex children, but which provides parents, carers, teachers, and health professionals with the insight, understanding, strategies, and techniques they need when living with and teaching this unique group of children. There probably are some "right" and "wrong" answers in this field, but ultimately what is right and wrong might only pertain to any given child and family. I do not personally believe that smacking is ever right, and I would propose that consistency is almost never wrong. I know that "love" is not enough, and that doing exactly what one is supposed to do day after day is too much to ask of anyone—parent/carer or child alike. On the other hand, child rearing is not about perfection; it is about doing the best that each of us can do. The chapters in this book do not talk about the right and wrong way of doing things. The material is designed to give ideas and examples of how one might approach a problematic situation, and then to draw upon those examples to formulate a programme of one's own.

About being adopted or in care

Daniel is a very attractive six-year-old who came to live with Shirley and Marcus, his prospective adoptive parents, three months before Shirley brought him to the clinic. Although he does not tell the therapist this, Daniel remembers the night the police broke into his mother's house and took his mother's boyfriend away. He knows he was afraid to go to sleep for days after that, always expecting the police to come again—and then they did: two of them, a woman and a man. They told Daniel and his older sister to get into the police car with them and the social worker and then they drove away. Daniel and Christie saw their mother once after that, but the social worker was with them, so no one talked or said very much. Daniel's mother hugged him and she was crying. Christie would not go near her mother and ignored Daniel. Christie and Daniel were placed in separate homes; Daniel does not know why. He missed his sister, whom he saw once a month at the Big Burger for about an hour during the next year. The foster carers were always with them, so they did not talk a lot together, but Daniel knew that Christie would not talk much anyway. When he asked her where their mother was, she told him to shut up. Daniel still worries about his mother all of the time.

Daniel was moved from his first foster home to another one because "I broke too many things in the first house." He says he has a lot of accidents but usually doesn't mean to break things. After another few months in the second foster home, he was moved to Shirley and Marcus's house. The social worker tells Daniel that he needs to "get adjusted" before she can arrange a date for him with his sister. Daniel doesn't know what getting adjusted actually means, so he is not sure what he is waiting for. He wants to visit with Christie and he wants to know where his mother is, because he worries about whether or not she is okay.

Almost all children come into care through the social service and the judicial systems. The majority of these children are under three years of age when they first enter care, with the average age of an adopted child being about four and a half years. A considerable number of young teenagers also enter the care system each year.

In England, in 2006, there were approximately 60,300 children in care, about 3,700 of whom were adopted (DfES, 2006). Sadly, however, adoption is rarely the next port of call for children who come into the care system. The unfortunate fact is that most children make numerous trips back home and out again—often going to different foster homes on each re-entry into care. While for some the voyage may be into what is labelled "short-term care", others are shipped from short-term to long-term care. The length of short- or long-term care can vary according to individual social service departments or private agencies. Only a relatively small number of children eventually journey into adoption. In this metaphor of travel, there is a kind of (e)motional sickness that inevitably takes hold on many of these young travellers.

In the plethora of early child development research, there is not a single piece of literature that says moving young children from home to home and carer to carer is a positive thing to do. Nevertheless, children in care are subjected to this experience repeatedly. It is little wonder, then, that these youngsters develop a wide range of psychosocial difficulties, "attachment issues" often being foremost among their sensitivities. Similarly, ADHD/ADD symptoms may be one of the many consequences that will be manifested in those whose early lives have been spent in chaotic environments.

Children who come into care almost never do so because of a one-off incident. More often than not, they enter the system after a long bout of dysfunction in their home environment. Many have been brought into care after having been rushed away from inadequate settings where it has been felt that protection of the child has become paramount, so the child often is not prepared for, or even talked to about, being taken away from his/her parent. Issues of attachment and separation that would have been fragile previously, suddenly become increasingly disturbed.

In her novel, *Latecomers* (1989), Anita Brookner writes about the sadness of a lost childhood:

> Both had been so deprived of childhood that in a sense they were both still waiting in the wings, unaware that, happy or unhappy, this stage must be passed, that beginnings are to a certain extent situated in limbo . . . [p. 125]

A significantly increasing number of children in the twentieth/twenty-first century have been adopted from overseas. "Non-domestically" adopted children tend to be quite a bit younger than domestic children, and they come through a very different network. In many developing countries, where poverty is so prevalent, infants are often left at orphanages or hospital doorsteps, or even on bridges, where mothers know that they will be found and picked up. These are absolutely destitute mothers who do not literally abandon their infants, but who leave them in obvious places in their hope of giving the child a better life. Contrary to the mother's hopes and expectations, though, many of these infants languish in poor, inadequate, institutionalized care for long periods of time before they become available for adoption, if that is, in fact, the destination for them. The scars of institutional life leave children highly at risk for a variety of developmental and emotional weaknesses, ADHD/ADD among them (Juffer & van Ijzendoorn, 2005; Rutter, 1998). Nevertheless, children from foreign countries are less frequently subjected to abject abuse and violence (even though serious malnutrition and neglect have very possibly been their experience), and they do tend to be adopted at younger ages than domestically adopted children, who experience years in and out of their own and other people's homes.

A substantial number of children, both domestically and non-domestically in care or adopted, are born to mothers exposed to malnutrition, extreme poverty, chaos, violence, and/or to parents having mental health vulnerabilities. In addition, substance affected parents are contributing to a growing population of children requiring out of home care. It is common knowledge that children of economically, socially, and emotionally impoverished families can be vulnerable to neurological, physiological, and developmental disorders. The result is that high numbers of children entering the care system are already fragile neurologically and emotionally. On the other hand, these same children are often unusually strong of nature and temperament because they have managed to survive untenable and extremely difficult situations.

Children come into the care system for a wide variety of reasons, but for all of these children, there is an interruption in the natural order of parenting, almost always as a result of the birth mother's/father's inability to provide a secure, healthy, safe environment for the child. Children thus enter care with experience of familial instability, fear, and hurt, but they also enter care with an astonishing ability to adapt to unpleasant situations. No matter what their age, they will have developed strategies to survive their previous experiences, and they will have organized patterns of behaving and thinking to accommodate moving into new living environments. While these behaviour patterns usually ensure the child's survival, they are often not socially acceptable behaviours and they rarely meet the expectations of the child's new carers.

Children who are survivors of long-term harm and trauma tend to lack empathy and social skills. Indeed, they often have survived either by becoming quite aggressive or by withdrawing. There is an apparent, but somewhat deceptive, resiliency in these children. It is a harsher, more rigid and less malleable resiliency than one would see in a child who is strong and independent because of a background ensuring trust, confidence, and security. Resiliency for the child in care usually means the ability to stay alive, but it has worked, and so this will not be behaviour that will be readily discarded.

On the other hand, and fascinatingly so, there certainly is a portion of adopted/looked after children who do bring with them rather astonishing resilience skills and a temperament that enables them to carry on with life in quite a reasonable manner. This group of children manages to negotiate day-to-day living in spite of deprivation and abuse that would have shattered most other youngsters. Probably, however, they are not children with ADHD/ADD, because the emotive and impulsive behaviour of the ADHD/ADD child does not lend itself to environmental or social adaptation.

Frequently, the troubled histories and compromised environments of children in care contribute to the child's keen alertness to danger, insecurity, violence, and inconsistency. These are children who hear a siren on the street a mile away, who worry about the sharp pencil lying on the desk next to them, who interpret a kind pat on the back as a potential threat ("She hit me first, so I had to hit her back"). They are the children who know exactly how much the dinner lady has given to the child in front of and behind them in the cafeteria queue, and they are acutely aware of how many balloons, or gold stars, or sweeties were given to every single child in class. Paying so much attention to their environmental surroundings inhibits them from being able to focus on their own self and being. While they know what everyone else is doing or supposed to do, they are equally vapid about a particular task or instruction required of them. Therefore, while these children have developed an acute sense of hyper-vigilance, they are inclined not to attend to those tasks which parents, carers, and teachers would like them to.

Jacob is a six-year-old who has been in three foster homes in the past four years. This is what he says about his day:

> When I wake up in the morning, I hear the baby next door crying, and that makes me scared, so I don't get dressed properly and then stupid Sam who shares my room always makes fun of me, so I have to get him out of my way, and then my foster mother comes in and says something that makes me think of other things—usually things about my baby sister because she is still at home with my mother and I don't know if my mum is drinking with that guy friend of hers or not. I think if my baby sister could come live with me, I could be better.

When children are removed from their homes, they are unfamiliar with alternative life-styles that might be presented to them by foster carers. All of us, as small children, know only what we have been exposed to, and we assume that our lives are typical of everyone else's. When we are very young, we have no basis of comparison. Since babies and young children use parents as role models, and since they have no ability to evaluate whether their parents' behaviours are good, bad, or neutral, they simply copy what they see and hear, and they make the necessary adaptations to adjust their feelings and responses to their environment. They also pick up the language they hear, again with no ability to determine whether this is proper language to use or not. When these children first move into a new home, they bring the emotions and behaviours of their history with them. They may be confused by the dramatically different atmosphere of the new home, and they tend to be completely unaware that their own behaviour might not be acceptable to their prospective care-takers. As a result, they spend a lot of time and energy trying to recreate situations that are familiar to them and that they know how to respond to or control, but again, the behaviours and language they use and what they are trying to create are not necessarily of a socially acceptable nature.

As an example, when food is rarely or very inconsistently available, children will quickly learn to steal, to hoard, to overeat, or to detach from their feelings of hunger. Almost all foster carers have had experiences with children who do all or any one of these things. Food can become a major source of dissention for a child and a foster carer, especially so if the carer has not been taught about this common characteristic of children coming into care. The child, however, will have no idea that he/she is behaving unusually or badly. The child is continuing to practise survival skills that have been highly beneficial in the past. Since trust has not previously been part of the equation in the child's relationships with adults, there is no reason for that child to believe the carer who says: "You don't have to eat too much now or hide food in your room because there will be tea later on and because you can always go to the kitchen and eat if you feel hungry." This is an entirely alien concept to the child who is used to going hungry because no food is available or allowed, or who has been promised food but then not had any.

Although food can be a source of aggravation to foster carers and adopters, it is mild compared to the more critically challenging behaviours that the looked after child may bring into the home. Children who are used to being abused frequently provoke abusive behaviour because they then feel they have a measure of control over it. A child who anticipates that mother will eventually scream and hit later in the evening (perhaps when she has been drinking too much), might consciously or unconsciously provoke mother to get angry when the child is prepared for the beating and feels that he/she can deal with it. It is scarier not to know when the beating may come than it is to cause it and be in control of it.

When children who have had these experiences come into families that do not smack or shout, they feel ill at ease and on their guard. Over and over again, they try to antagonize the parents/carers because they feel safe when they are in control and when they manage to re-establish an environment with which they are familiar. This oppositional and defiant behaviour on the part of the child is so difficult to deal with that adults can become exasperated enough to unintentionally create the precise situation that the child was trying to promote. Adopted/looked after children with ADHD/ADD are especially good at creating this atmosphere because children with attention deficits also need to live in rigid and predictable environments over which they feel they have control. Therefore, one part of the child may be creating the known atmosphere because that is what the ADHD/ADD factor is mandating, while another part of the child may be creating this same "known" environment for emotional reasons. Although we all feel safer when we are in control of ourselves, and ultimately that is surely the goal that parents/carers are hoping to instil in a child, the amount of energy that the ADHD/ADD adopted/looked after child spends maintaining the control panel for everything that goes on in his/her environment all day long can be very exhausting.

There are adopted and looked after children who do not behave this disruptively and who do manage to adapt satisfactorily to new homes and schools, but ADHD children are not known for their adaptability, so the adopted/looked after child who does show adaptation skills is probably not one who has ADHD.

Attention deficit hyperactivity disorder/ attention deficit disorder

> Daniel's disruptive, volatile nature, coupled with his inability to stay for any period of time with a game or toy or book, reflects the behaviour of most children with ADHD. Shirley finds him hard to please and difficult to satisfy. Marcus gets discouraged because playing with Daniel is not a lot of fun.
>
> Daniel, too, is frustrated living with his new parents. He doesn't understand Shirley's lack of appreciation for what he tries to do for her. Yesterday he stole a lipstick from the corner shop to give to Shirley, and instead of being pleased, she made him take it back. His birth mother would have smiled at him for that, even if her boyfriend would have smacked him across the face. Daniel was hurt that Shirley made him return the lipstick, so he broke her favourite flower vase and then screamed for a long time, and he wouldn't say he was sorry—because he wasn't.

The discussion surrounding ADHD/ADD in the last few decades has been diverse and often contentious. The ADHD/ADD literature is extensive, most of it originating in the USA and Australia, although, in recent years, numerous British and other European researchers have contributed substantially to the field. Unfortunately, this plethora of literature has only muddied the waters, with the result that anyone can pretty much substantiate any point of view regarding one's perspective on ADHD. Some would say that ADHD is the most controversial health issue of our time.

ADHD has probably been featured in more books, journals, popular magazines, scientific magazines, TV/radio programmes, schools, families, churches, playgrounds, chemists, and research laboratories nationally and internationally than has any other subject matter. Nevertheless, when one asks, "What is it?", there is little consensus as to an exact and reliable definition. Furthermore, the logical sequential question, "If you have it, what do you do about it?", elicits as many treatment measures as people who address the question.

Children with ADHD / ADD are sometimes depicted as children with neurobiological weaknesses and chemical disorders and / or with emotional, behavioural, and psychological impairments. Sometimes they are viewed as victims of poor parenting and / or as products of compromised environments. Like adopted / looked after children, ADHD / ADD youngsters can be labelled as "doomed" regardless of their environments, or as children who will be "just fine" if given the right environment.

Lloyd, Stead, and Cohen in *Critical New Perspectives on ADHD* (2006), argue that ADHD does not exist as a medical disorder, but only as a behavioural challenge. It is their view that parents are responsible for both creating and correcting ADHD behaviours. Although the book's introduction purports to take "a critical perspective on the growing phenomenon of ADHD", in fact, most of the chapters share the view that it is the systems surrounding the child that "are supporting and perpetuating the increasing diagnosis of ADHD and the resulting medicalisation of the behaviour of children" (p. 3). Several contributors to this book suggest that ADHD is not biologically or neurologically determined, but can be brought about by attributes of family and environment that may be associated with the behavioural characteristics of ADHD (e.g., Ongel, Chapter Seven).

On the other hand, *The Diagnostic and Statistical Manual of Mental Disorder (DSM IV)*, which is the "Michelin Guide" of psychiatric manuals, describes ADHD / ADD at length, detailing it as a "disruptive behavior disorder". Dr Russell Barkley, one of the original researchers into ADHD, continues to maintain that ADHD is "a developmental disorder of the ability to regulate behavior" (Barkley, 2000, p. 25).

In the middle, there are researchers such as Stein and Chowdhury who, in *Disorganized Children* (2006), point out that physicians have been trying to link behavioural and emotional difficulties with underlying neurological deficits for over 200 years, with a clinical description of ADHD first appearing in 1902 (p. 13). Stein and Chowdhury suggest that a spectrum of symptoms related to various emotional, behavioural, social, and educational impairments all fall onto a very broad continuum. Many of these symptoms and behaviours mirror those of ADHD.

For those who recognize ADHD/ADD as a neurodevelopmental disorder, there is much agreement about the symptoms. They concur that ADHD/ADD consists of problems with attention span, impulse control, distractibility, concentration, and regulation of mood. ADHD is frequently accompanied by learning disorders, although intelligence itself is not affected. (It is performance that is affected.) Chaotic parenting is seen as being detrimental for those who have ADHD/ADD, but is not viewed as a cause of the disorder. As poverty in and of itself is not seen as a reason for children to enter the care system, neither is poverty or one's mental health status seen as being a reason for having ADHD/ADD; but these are factors that might make it more difficult for a parent to deal with an ADHD/ADD child and which contribute to its lack of improvement. The situation in which both the child and the parent have ADHD/ADD presents a rather lethal combination for those families who have little emotional or practical support and for those parent–child relationships in which parenting skills are already fragile.

The uninhibited behaviour of ADHD children leads to impairment in how well rules and instructions can be understood, remembered, followed, and carried out. Their inability to control their behaviours, even when intellectually they know the rules, prevents them from making wise decisions, from keeping friends, from succeeding at school, and from getting along well at home or in the community. ADHD children exhibit behaviour that is too strong, too much, too "in-your-face". They are overly emotional and overly reactive. Children with ADD (no hyperactivity) can be too little of everything: oblivious, vague, "out-to-lunch", and enormously forgetful. ADHD and ADD children mean well, but cannot follow through, and this impedes their social and academic success. In fact, the formal criteria for ADHD/ADD require that symptoms must lead to "impairment of function", which is certainly the case for children suffering from this disorder (Barkley, 1996; Smart, 2003).

While one speaks of the "criteria" for ADHD/ADD, it must be remembered that there is not an absolute and definitive diagnosis of this condition. Unlike diabetes, chicken pox, or blindness, there is no laboratory test, X-ray or MRI that clearly defines and diagnoses ADHD/ADD. However, many professionals who admit they cannot clinically define ADHD still believe it exists. Most feel that there is a spectrum of disorders on a continuum that produce more or fewer ADHD/ADD characteristics, and when there are quite a number of these characteristic dysfunctions, ADHD/ADD behaviour seems to prevail. (Some of the characteristics themselves, however, are only labelled "disorders" subjectively, because many people would categorize high energy, the ability to multi-task, to see the big picture, and to have a broad range of interests as positive and enviable traits.) Moreover, ADHD/ADD is seen by clinicians as a neurological disorder, but one that is described in behavioural terms.

It is not clear whether there is an over-diagnosis or an under-diagnosis of children with ADHD/ADD. Girls are thought to be under-diagnosed because they do not as often display hyperactivity and are therefore left to sit quietly alone. About seven out of ten children diagnosed with ADHD/ADD are boys. Depending upon what one reads and how updated the information is, in the USA the percentage of school age children with ADHD/ADD is often estimated to be somewhere between 3% and 6% (Barkley, 2000; American Academy of Child and Adolescent Psychiatry: Facts for Families, 2004), while in the UK it is more usually estimated to be 3–5% (www.nice.org.uk, 2006). Some researchers feel that Europeans are more reluctant to diagnose ADHD/ADD, while others contend that their criteria differ, and thus the percentages of children with ADHD/ADD are seen to be different. Among adoptees, it is agreed that the rate of ADHD/ADD jumps to 20–30% in both the UK and the USA (Silver, 1999). Again there are no definitive reasons for this, although heredity is assumed to play a large role.

Much recent research does support the belief that there is a heredity component involved in ADHD. Indeed, in reviewing contemporary research, one finds many allusions to the heritability of ADHD/ADD (Barkley, 2000; Deutsch et al., 1982; Faraone & Doyle, 2001). Biederman et al. (1992) have written that genetic analysis of twin and adoption studies suggest that there is a heritable component in some children and adults. Some studies suggest that as many as 40% of children with ADHD will have a biological parent with ADHD—usually the father. Sprich, Biederman, Crawford, Mundy, and Faraone (2000) found that, in a family study of adopted children with ADHD, the rate of ADHD in adoptive parents and their adopted children was low, but the rate of adoptees with ADHD biological parents was significantly higher. Moreover, this study found high rates of mood and anxiety disorders among the biological parents of ADHD adoptees, but not among the adoptive parents.

Dr Paul Carter, among others, feels that 70–90% of ADHD is inherited, but Dr Carter describes it in terms of "rolling the dice". He says that "how the genetics roll out" can be seen in the first eighteen days of life, but it takes another two years to know how the neuroanatomy will be influenced by the environment (Carter, 2006). Carter suggests that inadequate parenting and stressed environmental conditions can exacerbate a vulnerable neurobiological system, whereas a strong, positive, loving and attentive environment is influential in helping to minimize the potential disturbances. Golding (2004) too would concur that some children who struggle with inconsistently available parents develop patterns of behaviour that exhibit anxiety and ambivalent relationships characterized by aggression, attention difficulties, impulsivity, and hyperactivity: all characteristics of the ADHD child. Certainly, this has implications for adopted and looked after children.

The overlap of ADHD/ADD and adoption/fostering

> "Concentration is good in exams, bad in orange juice" (Guy Browning, the *Guardian*, September 2006).

Although ADHD appears to have a genetic basis, other factors influence the development of the disorder, and it is this "influence possibility" that confuses the cause of ADHD for so many people. While supporters of ADHD/ADD as a neurological disorder will focus on brain development and other medical conditions that can precipitate or confound ADHD, others will stress that it is the environment that aggravates or inhibits attention behaviours. Prenatal drug or alcohol exposure, prematurity, lead poisoning, and other similar conditions are all thought to be able to put a child at risk for ADHD (Adesman, 2006; Nigg, 2006). These are also conditions that often are part and parcel of the looked after child's environment and that contribute to a child being taken into care in the first place.

Many therapists purport that for adopted / looked after children, the added childhood task of trying to make sense of altered life circumstances influences the child's emotional stability and learning style. When infants and toddlers have needed to spend their early lives concentrating on survival and self-protection, their focus of attention becomes narrow and exclusive. This ultimately will have implications for how their brains develop.

As a result of neurological under-development, many adopted / looked after children suffer from internal dysregulation and an inability to manage their feelings, their belongings, their lives. Although they have not learned to trust adults and therefore do not comply with much of what is asked of them, they are nevertheless dependent upon these adults to provide stability and regularity on a daily basis. Like children with ADHD / ADD, adopted / looked after children flounder in tumultuous waves of disorganisation and dysfunction, but are desperate for that seemingly illusive gold ring which will provide them with a calm sea of predictability and consistency.

In one of the very few studies of ADHD and adoption, Simmel, Brooks, Barth, and Hinshaw (2001) investigated the rates of symptoms for specific externalizing behavioural disorders (ADHD and Oppositional Defiant Disorder) among a large sample of adopted youth. Their aim was to identify key risk factors that may predispose adopted youth to adverse behavioural, emotional and educational outcomes and to ascertain the impact of these difficulties on the youths' current functioning. In their study, pre-adoption abuse and neglect, as well as the age of placement in the adoptive home, appeared to be influential in the child's likelihood of having ADHD symptoms.

The combination of being in care or being adopted and of having attention disorders requires the intervention and co-operation of many adults if the child is to make improvements in his / her social-emotional-behavioural and academic careers. All of these professionals and carers need to be willing to think broadly and laterally so that a flexible, but consistent approach can be maintained. Medical professionals need to be thinking about trauma and its effects, while mental health professionals must not rule out the neuro-biological factors that can be involved. Both health and mental health providers must take into account the quality of care and the continuity of care for each individual child (Selwyn & Quinton, 2004; Silver, 1999).

Educational psychologists, physical and occupational therapists are an important part of this multi-modal team because all aspects of a child's history and current functioning must be well evaluated. Everyone will want to consider the possibilities of developmental issues such as learning disabilities, auditory processing difficulties, mood disorders or other dysfunctions that can occur either in conjunction with ADHD or without ADHD. It has been found that many ADHD/ADD children have co-morbid learning disorders that need to be addressed independently from their attentional difficulties. Attending to a speech and language disorder, for example, might not just improve the speech/language difficulty, but also, it may help to reduce the behaviours that have appeared to be ADHD characteristics. The treatment approach to a speech difficulty in and of itself, however, is different from methods used to aid a child with attention disorders so it is important to be sure that one knows what one is treating. On the other hand, if the child has ADHD in addition to the speech problem, the treatment will need to take that into consideration as well. This is a good example of why there are no easy answers in this field and why one difficulty can so easily complicate another.

As has been pointed out above, some children coming into the care system may have ADHD/ADD innately or genetically, and many others will appear to have the condition because their behaviours and emotions are impaired and they will display symptoms similar to those of the ADHD/ADD child. Some of these "disorganized," (Stein and Chowdhury, 2006), "unconventional" (Comfort, 1992), "out of sync" (Stock-Kranowitz, 2005) children (who may or may not be children in care), sometimes encompass a wide range of well-established neurological disorders that are similar to those described above for children being assessed for ADHD. These can be specific learning disorders, or they can be emotional and behavioural difficulties. Smith's 2001 investigations in Britain "indicated that nearly half of the children who had observable soft signs of neurological symptoms at age five had been diagnosed with learning disabilities by age ten," (quoted in Lavoie, 2006, p.13). In the same vein, adopted/looked after children may display the emotional and behavioural untidiness frequently manifested by children with ADHD. Many children in the care system and some who are thought to have ADHD do not fully meet the criteria of any one specific diagnosis, but they do suffer from the hidden handicaps that can impair their daily functioning and that impact significantly upon their families, carers and teachers (Brodzinsky & Schechter, 1990; Comfort, 1997).

Some difficulties that both ADHD/ADD and adopted/looked after children encounter are described in the points listed under the heading below, which are then explained in greater detail. Although many parents might find their children fall into one or several of these categories, it is unlikely that the normally developing child will be as pervasively and consistently affected by all of these disorders as frequently as is the ADHD/ADD adopted/looked after child.

What ADHD/ADD and adopted/looked after children have trouble doing

- Concentrating.
- Filtering out extraneous information.
- Planning/reflecting.

Concentrating

ADHD/ADD children are unable to keep their minds in control without learning how to do so and without a lot of practice. (Reading high interest books, stringing beads, doing puzzles, following recipes are examples of fun ways to practise these skills.)

Filtering information

They have difficulty filtering out irrelevant stimuli and focusing on the important task or information. Distractions of sounds, sights, smells, and ideas can get in their way. This is true for ADHD / ADD children and for adopted / looked after children independently. The combination of the two is fuel for the fire.

Planning/reflecting

Children with ADHD / ADD do not know how to organize, plan, and think about the course of action. Typically, they do not reflect upon their actions or make revisions in their plan of action. Many parents / carers and teachers try to work with charts and organizational tools to help children to: "Stop, Think, Act, Evaluate, Revise;" but these meet with varying success since it is hard for the child to take the required time to focus on and carry out this process.

What ADHD/ADD adopted/looked after children may experience

- Tiredness.
- Impulsivity.
- Mood control and difficulties with self regulation.
- Lack of gratification.
- Social isolation.
- Lowered self esteem.

Tiredness

It is thought that children with ADHD are actually tired. Their hyperactivity is their way of keeping themselves awake. Extra sleep would help, but they rarely do sleep much or for very long periods of time, so they are always tired.

Acting impulsively

These children are very poor at waiting, going slowly, taking turns, contemplating. They often act without thinking first. Weak internal regulation is reflected in their inability to stop themselves and to take control of their actions. Acting on impulse (gut-reaction) may have frequently contributed to the safety and survival of the child in care. This child's past experience (which was life-saving) will reinforce his/her inclination to continue to act this way. The ADHD child may realize that his/her impulsivity got him/her into trouble, but feels that there was no available control button to turn off the action.

Regulating moods

ADHD/ADD children are unstable in managing their feelings and emotional responses. Their moods tend to change quickly and unpredictably, and they have little control over this seesaw of emotion. Mood swings are scary for the person experiencing them and challenging for those in charge of that individual. Whether neurologically and/or emotionally based, the regulation of mood often requires medical or professional intervention.

Feeling satisfied/gratified

Children with these disorders always have a sense of needing something they do not have: constantly wanting more or something different; forever searching for a new source of stimulation, but nothing ever quite satisfies. This is an enormously difficult trait for both the child and the parent/carer as no one feels he or she can make the situation better. The ADHD/ADD child loves distractions, but functions best when hyper-focused. This same child seeks stimulation to ward off boredom, but over-stimulation is also what he/she suffers from. The novelty of a new toy or activity is very short-lived (often the toy ends up being broken). The child who has been traumatized may not trust any new situation or change of routine, so does not accept it, and ADHD/ADD children are very poor at transitions; yet children with either of these disorders feel unsatisfied if the situation stays the same.

Social isolation/lowered self esteem

These children have difficulty in making and keeping friends: they do not understand how to play with others or to join groups; they are unable to focus on any one interest long enough to engage with peers in games or sports or to share hobbies and leisure activities; they feel bad because no one wants to be their friend. Adopted/looked after children have so many secrets to keep, and their backgrounds rarely coincide with other children around them. They know that others do not/will not understand how they feel or think. Impulsively, ADHD/ADD adopted/looked after children might say more than they want to, revealing parts of their lives that result in their becoming targets for teasing and bullying. They often isolate themselves or become bullies, which automatically separates them from most of their peers. Not being understood or liked by others, they feel even worse about themselves. It is hard for them to believe or trust the person who says something nice to, or about, them, so they shrug the person off, alienating themselves even further.

Characteristics of young adopted/looked after children who might have ADHD/ADD

0–2 years

- They sleep, wake, and feed in a very disorganized fashion.
- They are unable to calm or soothe themselves.
- They do not stay with any activity for even a few minutes.
- They do not connect with an adult or peer for an age-related expected period of time.

2–6 years

- They continue to have trouble with sleeping, eating, and playing.
- They do not relate to others with any predictability.
- They do not know when or how to say or do what is appropriate or acceptable.
- They have trouble organizing their thoughts and ideas so do and say things erratically.
- They manifest vast and quickly changing mood states.
- They do not think before doing something, and often have many accidents because of this.

* * *

The relationship between adoption/being looked after and ADHD/ADD is further complicated because adoption/being looked after is neither a condition nor a disorder. One does not "treat" adoption. Nevertheless, as is indicated above, some of the risk factors for coming into the care system are the same as the risk factors for having the "condition" of ADHD/ADD. Moreover, if a child already does have ADHD/ADD, living in disorganized households and being moved from home to home can only serve to aggravate the situation.

If parents of children with ADHD were not disorganized before, they most certainly will feel discombobulated by adding an ADHD child to their home—regardless of whether the child is biologically theirs or not. ADHD behaviour is hard for anyone to live with, whether at home or in the classroom. Often parents feel inadequate and unfulfilled. The constant disorganization, inattention, impulsivity, distractibility, day-dreaming, and arguing of the ADHD/ADD child can quickly wear them down. Thus, while the link between being fostered/adopted and having ADHD/ADD is not a clear one, "the correlation between ADHD and adoption is undeniable" (Richard Lavoie in conversation, 2006).

A mother of three biological sons who adopted two young boys when her birth children were almost grown, wrote in her diary, and told me: "I always thought I was a pretty good mother until these two little boys came into our lives. I had brought up sons, and know the difficulties that rambunctious, active, hungry, academically challenged boys can present; but never had I dreamed of the differences in my older sons and these boys. I don't even know how to explain why or what is so hard about them, but it just seems like everything. Nothing is ever right or smooth or rational."

Children presenting with disorganized styles, hyperactivity, and impulsivity are "accused" of being attention seekers. Indeed, seeking attention is exactly what they are doing, because they are in desperate need of attracting a consistent and reliable adult. Since they are poor at internal regulation, they need the stability of an outside person to help them to manage even the most mundane of daily living routines. Both ADHD/ADD children and children in the care system have developed these strategies, consciously or unconsciously, so that they can acquire the attention of adults who will scaffold and support their shaky framework.

A foster carer says: "Bonnie's teacher is constantly complaining that Bonnie needs her every second of the day—as if I don't already know that!—but it is true, she does need her (and me), all of the time, so I don't know what to tell the teacher any more. The teacher says I have to tell Bonnie to stop interrupting and stop asking for so much attention all of the time, but if it were that easy to do, this wouldn't be the problem that it is."

As is seen in the above example, the manifestations of a child's need for attention is reflected by parental complaints that the child requires constant input for everything, and often seems to "purposefully" do things wrong so as to acquire additional adult attention. These are the children who forget their lunch, don't remember to bring home school notices, leave their gym kits in the car, cannot organize their own play activities, and so forth. Teachers are constantly frustrated by children with attention problems because they do not remember where they left their homework; they never have a sharpened pencil—probably not any pencil; they cannot tolerate any change in the school routine; they are unable to follow directions, and they ask a million questions all day long. In this way, and because they feel misunderstood, emotionally alone, and inadequate, both ADHD/ADD and adopted/looked after children persist in their daily search to be found.

Unfortunately, most of our conversations and a great body of research work tend to focus on the negative aspects of ADHD/ADD children and adopted/looked after children, two groups that can often be one and the same group. Perhaps it would be helpful if there were more attention paid to the positive factors found in either or both of these groups so that we could learn more about what does work and if it is teachable to those who are still struggling. It is true that these children and their carers and teachers have a hard row to hoe, but there is also sometimes a humour or a breakthrough that can be quite charming and delightful, and one that is well worth noting. When caught in a good moment, many parents of adopted children with attention problems have been able to extol the virtues of their creative and sparky children. Indeed, these children can be inventive, amusing, charming, and totally engaging children at times, and we must not lose sight of that if we are to foster their achievement. (As it is known that many ADHD individuals share common characteristics with corporate executives and successful entrepreneurs (Kirby & Honeywood, 2007), it would be a shame to overlook or to discount the talents that these children display early on.)

One must concentrate, too, on the enormous resiliency that so many adopted/looked after children show us in their daily lives. I have found that this inner strength can be contagious. Siblings in families of children with difficult or disabling conditions often emerge as amazingly strong and competent young adults with empathy and sensitivity that is extraordinary. Teachers who learn from the children in their classroom will be better equipped to work with next year's student who is ADHD/ADD adopted/looked after, and so the cycle moves on.

CHAPTER TWO

Understanding the effects of maltreatment on early brain development and the consequences for ADHD/ADD and adopted/looked after children

> Christie sinks into her own quiet reveries, remembering the days when she would try to hide her brother from her mother's boyfriend. Christie was six at that time, Daniel not yet three. Sometimes she hid Daniel in the closet and other times she made him stay outside in the garage, even though it was cold and wet out there. She rubs her fingers over the scar on her own arm from the day the boyfriend found Daniel in the cupboard and beat Christie up for hiding him. Then the boyfriend was in her room that night and got into her bed. She tries to think about what happened next, but all she hears in her head is Daniel screaming—or maybe it was she who was screaming. Christie doesn't know where her mother was that night, and never allowed herself to "see" her mother again. Christie doesn't like to talk because she is afraid her voice might scream, so she stays quiet and blocks out much of what goes on around her.

In recent years, the focus on both adopted / looked after children and on ADHD / ADD has been very much influenced by developing research on early brain development. Investigators in ADHD have focused attention on the neurobiology of the disorder and adoption studies have centred much of their attention on the effects of abuse and neglect on the developing brain during infancy and early childhood (National Clearing House on Child Abuse and Neglect Information, 2001). The research is providing biological explanation for what practitioners had been describing previously in psychological, emotional, and behavioural terms. Although there is still much to be learned about the brain, and newly unfolding information may yet alter our conceptions of how both genetics and injury to the brain could affect a child's development, it is currently proposed that the neonate is highly influenced by what happens in utero. The infant's neurological condition can then be improved or jeopardized dramatically, depending upon environmental input, in the next three years (at which point the brain will have acquired 90% of its ultimate size). Shonkoff and Phillips (2000) indicate that there is abundant evidence from the behavioural and neurobiological sciences that documents a wide range of environmental threats that can significantly affect the early childhood years and beyond.

Pertinent to the topic of ADHD/ADD in adopted/looked after children is the finding that the brains of abused and neglected children are not as well integrated as the brains of non-abused children. Abused and neglected children have smaller *corpus callosum* than non-abused children, and abused/neglected children have poorly integrated cerebral hemispheres (Becker-Weidman, 2007). This helps to explain why abused and neglected children have significant difficulties with emotional regulation, integrated functioning, and social development. Moreover, MRI samples of ADHD children have found "significantly smaller prefrontal lobe and striatal regions in these children" (Barkley, 2006, p. 33), which supports the view that ADHD involves impairments in the development of the brain.

Fugard, in his novel, *Tsotsi* (1983), beautifully described how the older child who has been neurologically affected by an inadequate upbringing might feel inside of himself:

> His second rule . . . was never to disturb his inward darkness with the light of a thought about himself or the attempt at a memory . . . There was only a limited area that he controlled absolutely. The vaster regions of it operated regardless of him, sometimes running against his purpose. [p. 36]

Although the neurobiology of ADHD/ADD adopted/looked after children is critically important to their growth and development, it is certainly beyond the parameters of this book to delve into neurological or psychological explanations of how the brain develops or operates. On the other hand, it is useful to have a cursory understanding of what can happen when the brain is not given all of the chances it needs to mature properly. The neurodevelopmental framework of children who come into care is important to consider because these children are exposed to more risk factors, both before and after birth, thereby creating increased vulnerabilities for a multitude of problems, not the least of which could be attention deficits.

The developing brain is in the process of growing and pruning its neurons, much as one would do in cultivating one's garden. If flowers are to blossom, they need to be fairly weed-free; they need to be fertilized; they need to be attended to and talked to, and they require a basic amount of fundamental care. The flower cannot bloom if there are too many other roots pulling the nutrients away from it.

This is also what happens in the infant's developing brain. In a healthy family, the growth and pruning process happens quite spontaneously because even very basic, non-abusive parenting tends to provide a fertile enough environment in which the brain can prosper. Parents and carers who are attuned to small children will meet their physical and emotional needs by becoming aware of ("reading") and responding to the baby's cries and pleasures, by chatting with the infant, by providing appropriate stimulation and by forming an engagement with the baby. Like the garden flower, the child will be fed and watered, and this is healthy neurological food.

Babies whose care-givers can meet their needs on emotional and social levels, who respond in an appropriate manner to the sensory needs of the infant, and who are engaged in sensitive interactions, will have a different early experience from those in families who over-stimulate or who neglect or abuse the baby. Some babies, whose neonatal experience is hampered by drug-exposure, prematurity, birth defects, or neurological impairments, find it harder to adapt to their surroundings. These can be children who are more difficult to parent because they may not be easily soothed or understood and they may be unresponsive to their carers. As a result, babies who are harder to care for and less satisfying to carers are often more vulnerable to abuse and neglect.

Although the infant described above finds it more difficult to form attachments, which in turn makes it harder for the parent/carer to bond with the child, the brain itself can be quite brilliant at adapting to its surroundings. In making this adaptation, the brain will adjust itself to a negative environment just as easily as to a positive one. Resilience in the face of stress is adaptive mental health, but the materials required for this adaptation may take away from, or interfere with, the normal growth process of the child's developing brain. Therefore, children in violent, abusive, or otherwise dysfunctional households risk losing certain cortical pathways and/or neuron synapses in the neurobiological structuring and development of their brain. It can happen that these children become overly focused on maintaining the early neuron pathways that concentrate on survival and on self-protection. They may also be turning off those pathways that tell them other things they need to know, thus not allowing the brain to develop the more complex cortical system that contributes to how we modulate our affect and control our impulsivity, for example.

One way in which we might recognize these shortcomings in ADHD/ADD adopted/looked after children is by their inability to identify their own internal needs. Infants must learn to acknowledge signs indicating that they are hungry, cold, wet, hurt, or tired, but an infant who does not have these needs met by a reliable outside source, may get stuck right in this primitive state of survival. If these needs are sometimes, but not predictably or reliably met, it is possible for the child to shut down sensory recognition of hunger or cold or any other feeling-state. Children in traumatic circumstances may have developed brain patterns that are so entrenched that the brain no longer sends feeling messages to the rest of the body. In these situations, the children don't "feel" or don't know what they feel—a complaint often voiced amongst foster carers and adopters about children in their care. These are children who have "turned off", because why would one keep pressing the switch if the light never goes on?

Countless carers of looked after and adopted children despair about the lack of awareness of and responsiveness to the carer or to others. The following remarks are only a few of those that could easily fill a book by themselves.

"I ask him if he is hungry, but he always says no."

"Even when she hurts herself, she doesn't cry or seek out sympathy from anyone around her."

"She looks straight through me as though there is nothing there."

"He never pays attention to a word I say."

Some children, perhaps those of a hardier temperament, who have put feelings behind them, are able to skip the first developmental hurdle and move on to the next one. Needless to say, this is a dangerous jump, and a child who is forced to take such a big leap will be jeopardizing the subsequent stages of his/her growth and development.

Children who have been traumatized tend to live in a state of neurological disorder with an abnormally high sense of hyperarousal, over-reactivity (fight or flight) and little ability to self-soothe. They tend not to be able to make an accurate or appropriate assessment of a situation, so behave according to their own internal needs and perceptions rather than to the reality of the situation. These are children with whom it is very difficult to make an attachment because their internal world operates so differently from the expectations of others.

The young infant requires good bonding and attachment experiences in order to achieve optimal brain development. Secure attachment is really the base of all social–emotional and behavioural growth because a sound link with a loving and reliable adult provides the child not only with a secure and trustworthy foundation on which to grow, but also with a model for future relationships and interactions. Without this foundation of trust, the child's successful development can be seriously impeded. Severe neglect and the absence of being cared for properly can cause various degrees of brain deficits and behaviour problems in maltreated children. Other aspects of the child's make-up and the environment in which he/she is living combine to influence how adaptively the child manages to cope. The interplay of parent and child and of the environment and the child can never be underestimated because it is that dyad and the individual temperaments and qualities each brings to the relationship that will facilitate or jeopardize growth and development in both the carer and the child. Neither the strong-willed nor the more malleable child is an entity unto herself, because the personality and temperament of the carer will add to or detract from either child's chance of getting on in life.

Even with relatively significant neurological disorders or maladaptive environments, some infants and babies manage to do better than others. How useful it would be if we knew why, but individual resiliency is not well understood and can only be evaluated within the context of the environment.

Fascinated by an early adolescent whose life, until she was adopted at eight years of age, was filled with neglect and deprivation, I once asked her how it was that she coped so well at school and at home. Her response: "I just blow a lot of things off." How she managed to do that was a mystery both to her and to me, but it was all that she knew how to understand or verbalize about her own behaviour.

To return to the garden metaphor and the growing of neurological synapses, a substance-abusing parent is unlikely to be sufficiently attending to the plant she has created. Alcohol and drug abuse in pregnancy can alter the way the cortex develops, as these substances will reduce the number of neurons produced. Neurobiological problems, such as difficulties with attention, memory, problem solving, and abstract thinking may result. These difficulties will come into the world with the child, but further social and emotional dysfunctions are likely to emerge if the infant stays in an abusive, neglectful environment. As has been said, many children who enter the care system have come from substance abusive pregnancies, so it is not surprising that some of these children will experience attention difficulties.

During the nine months of pregnancy, the neurological system develops from the bottom up, so that the cortex of the brain is one of the last pieces to come together in this process. Serotonin is a chemical that is required by cortex neurons for their metabolism, and the amount of serotonin in the cortex seems to have some influence on the way ADHD/ADD adopted/looked after children function. Although ADHD individuals appear to have too little serotonin, children in care who have been exposed to repeated stress and trauma seem to have too much of it. Thus, children with attention deficits might have too little serotonin to maximize their ability to cope with stressful life events. At the same time, children in the care system, who may have too much serotonin running around their nervous system, may have desensitized their neurons, which also leads to poor ability to cope with life's daily challenges. Where, one might rightfully wonder, does this leave the ADHD/ADD adopted/looked after child?

How parents, carers and the environment influence brain development

Most children who enter the care system will have lived initially with a birth parent who verbalizes (and means!) that she wants to parent well and that she loves her baby. The problem is that this parent is often consumed by other needs that assume priority over her child. This leads to inconsistent parenting and an unreliable home environment, so that at times the infant will be talked to and played with (possibly in excess of what the small baby can actually tolerate) and sometimes the baby will be completely ignored. Usually, too, the parent plays with the child on the adult's whim and desire rather than in conjunction with what the baby may be ready for. When a baby wants and needs to sleep, it is not a comfortable time for her to be thrown into the air or poked and played with. On the other hand, when a baby is awake and aroused, he does need the attention and involvement of his care-takers. Stimulation at the wrong time is an interference with body and mood stability, and either the lack of stimulation or the presence of chaotic stimulation can be responsible for interrupting healthy child development.

When parents with mental health difficulties or substance abuse problems are unable to offer the child a positive growth-producing environment, the child's brain maturation is unlikely to achieve the desired goals. The garden does not flourish under these circumstances, and is in need of a new gardener. Clearly, substance abuse and parenting are not compatible. Infants and toddlers born into chemically dependent families frequently suffer poor physical health and they are exposed to social and emotional challenges that are better coped with in later life.

Once again, Brookner, in her novel *Latecomers* (1989), describes this succinctly: "In everything pertaining to his past, he was prerational. He possessed inexhaustible reserves of terror, or rather of horror, which could be, and were, activated in defiance of his conscious will" (p. 145).

When parents with addiction problems are unable to care for their children because they are easily distracted themselves by their own mental health difficulties or their chemical dependency, they not only pass on risk for neurological disorders, but they also provide an inadequate model for the child who is trying to make sense of the world around him. An infant who is exposed to a distractible model, and/or an infant who suffers from an impaired nervous system, is unlikely to learn much about stress reduction and relaxation techniques. Infants and young children in substance abusive homes are observed to be those who cry frequently and are unable to soothe themselves or allow others to soothe them. As their internal thermostats do not operate reliably, these children often have eating and sleeping disturbances and depression is not uncommon (Lowry, 2007; Perry, 2001; Perry, Runyan, & Sturges, 1998). Of course, this makes them hard-to-care-for babies, leaving a distressed infant or toddler in the hands of an equally distressed parent. While all families experience disorder and exhaustion some of the time, most do not live continuously with the utter despair that both mother and child must feel throughout the day and night when neither is able to calm either herself or the other.

Disorganized infants face a difficult dilemma because their source of security is also their source of distress. These are children who manifest significant attachment problems, and are often those taken into care. It has been well documented that impoverished attachment is linked to poor outcomes in a number of areas:

- managing affect;
- impulsivity;
- low self-esteem;
- difficulty with empathy;
- fragile social-emotional and physical health;
- diminished ability to self-regulate;
- learning disorders.

Children whose attachment ties have been severed can suffer from all or any of the above. They are special needs youngsters who require special and extraordinary care-giving and teaching.

Ironically, children with quite significant attention difficulties might experience these same feelings, not because their parents did not provide a warm and loving family environment, but because the child was unable to perceive or make use of what was being offered. Since many children with ADHD / ADD do not read social and emotional cues accurately, they frequently have trouble with interpreting their environment in the same manner that most others do. They may interpret a mother's smile as "mother is laughing at / making fun of me", or they may perceive a warm pat on the back as "dad is always hitting me". Similarly, a well-meaning teacher may approach the child's desk to help a child with a difficult task, but that child, who is on constant alert to the dangers of adults who approach too closely, may lash out aggressively and unexpectedly. Children who misperceive what is going on around them struggle to fit in and to make coherent sense of their world, complicating their own lives as well as the lives of those who are trying hard to help them.

Not infrequently, adopted / looked after children or ADHD / ADD children, or both, are found to have processing difficulties. Since their minds have not been able to stay still long enough to hear or see information, to take it in, to process it, and to turn it out meaningfully, they are not children who take responsibility for their actions or understand their role in events. Sequentially, things did not happen for them in the same way they did for others—their leaping minds probably missed out a step or did not slow down enough to reflect upon what was happening—so they interpret the situation differently. It is easy for these children to blame someone else for what happened because they truly do not appreciate that they had an active role in what was going on. This is the "he hit me first" scenario, because the ADHD / ADD adopted / looked after child just does not recognize that it was he who initiated the pushing and shoving, the irritated smirks, the unkind language. All he knows or remembers is that someone hit him.

As is seen above, when the brain has not developed as it should, children may have trouble managing some or many aspects of how they feel and learn and behave. These children may over-react to relatively minor issues, or they may not respond at all and go into a "frozen" state. The psycho-emotional effect of trauma can be as harmful and long lasting as are the specific neurological outcomes. Heineman (1998) emphasizes that

> Neither a single beating nor a single sexually abusive act are isolated intrapsychic incidents; they continue to influence the course of the child's development. Abused children suffer the effects of mistreatment for many, many years and in complex ways. [p. 19]

As these emotions may ebb and flow or arise almost without warning, the individual's behaviour or emotional outburst may appear to others to be irrational, but to the individual who is reliving the trauma, it is very real and intense. A child in the care system or one who has been adopted (even years after the adoption took place) who is trying to work out and deal with the shadows of the past, may act in ways that mirror the behaviours of an ADHD child. The similarity of their inability to focus, their impulsivity, their mood swings, and their insatiability clothe them like costumes for the roles that each is acting. Given different circumstances, who knows what part the child in care may have played.

It has already been pointed out that substance abuse is harmful to the neonate and to the developing child. Alcohol, cocaine, and methamphetamine exposure *in utero* have been shown to result in babies with low birth weight, neurobehavioural difficulties, foetal alcohol disorders, and failure to thrive, among other dysfunctions (Diamond-Berry, 2007). Yet, substance abuse is certainly not the only cause for neonate vulnerability.

Equally, malnutrition, maternal trauma, and poor physical or mental health are among the many precursors of neurological disorders and physiological difficulties that can affect a child's development. There are large numbers of children who come into the care system who have been exposed to pre- and post-natal malnutrition—especially those youngsters who have been adopted from overseas. Malnutrition is not actually a complete entity in and of itself, though, because some pregnant women may lack particular vitamins or minerals while others may simply lack adequate amounts of food. Depending upon what aspects of nutrition have been compromised, certain neurological and physiological consequences may occur. For example, even many healthy and well-fed pregnant women are given supplemental iron, since iron deficiency is known to result in motor and cognitive delays. Lack of iron during the pregnancy can also later affect a child's social relationships and it can lead to depression and to problems with attention.

Another neurological characteristic shared by adopted/looked after and ADHD/ADD children is poor internal modulation, or an inability to regulate their emotions, moods, and desires. Mood regulation is a task of very early childhood, and it is especially difficult to regain this ability once it has been overstepped. Unfortunately, lacking control of one's self is quite scary. While there are always extenuating circumstances, most of us know how we will act or respond to relatively mundane situations, and as parents/carers, most of us have a fairly good idea of what our children are likely to do. This is not true for the child or the parent of one whose internal regulation system does not work reliably. For the ADHD/ADD adopted/looked after child, the arc of the swing can be quite large and, equally, can plunge from high to low, or vice versa, with amazing rapidity. Children chase their own emotions around this playground with the same frenetic weariness that their carers do, but neither is usually very successful in capturing stability without therapeutic intervention.

For children in care who are always (rightfully) worried about being moved to a new home or new school, the emotional factors associated with changes in placements and separation from family put heavy demands on an already weakened system. For ADHD/ADD children, whose neurotransmitters are not connecting or sending stable messages, there is also a hefty demand placed on a fragile system. Their inability to self-regulate may cause them to exaggerate their thoughts and emotions and may lead them to act inappropriately, or in an extreme or outrageous manner that clearly reflects how out of control they really are.

ADHD/ADD children who have started life in a more stable environment have an improved chance in their neurological garden growing. For them, the appropriate neonatal reflexes will have disappeared because they were no longer required. In the meantime, more advanced and complicated pathways were able to start developing, leading the baby to explore and adapt to his home and family. Although the ADHD/ADD child may struggle within, and may not always have perceived correctly what was on offer, at least this child has had the benefit of an environment that is not also working against him (although his own perception of it may be). This is a child who will have been attended to in a good enough manner, even though his particular needs may not have been specifically addressed. While the youngster may still experience difficulties with self regulation, with focusing on a task, with hyperactivity, or the myriad other characteristics that describe the ADHD/ADD child, at least he will not have been deterred in his neurological growth by extreme trauma, abuse, or neglect.

On the other hand, like children in care, the ADHD/ADD child who is unable to regulate moods and responses will tend to either remain hyper-aroused or dissociated at least some of the time. Also like the child in care, sometimes they do both of these erratically and unpredictably. Equally, both groups can be worried and depressed out of fear of not keeping up with their peers and not being understood at home and in the classroom.

> Luke is ten years old and has ADHD. He goes to respite foster care once a month for a weekend because he lives with a disabled single mother who manages fairly well, but is easily worn out by her four children and her own physical difficulties. Luke likes home and foster care, but described his worries about being in school this way:
>
> "I normally like science classes quite a bit, but when the teacher began talking about the fish in the ocean, I immediately started thinking about the trip my foster family took me on to the sea last summer. I remembered that I caught a large tuna. Thinking of that made me hungry, and I wondered if Mum put a tuna sandwich in my lunch box today. I was so anxious to eat the tuna sandwich that I just got out of my seat and headed toward the locker where we keep the packed lunches. When the teacher asked what I thought I was doing, it puzzled me, and then I got scared because the class started laughing and I didn't know what to say or do. I often get distracted like that. One thing makes me think of another, and then I am off."

As an aside: most ADHD/ADD children of normal cognitive ability in most families know and understand the home expectations and the school rules. They pretty much know what they are supposed to do and not do in their homes and families and in the classroom. Not being able to control their impulses, though, these children tend to act before thinking and impulsively do whatever happens to be on their mind. On the other hand, children brought up in dysfunctional environments and those who have had repetitive moves may not even know or understand what behaviour is expected of them. Regardless of the child's cognitive ability, his lifestyle may not have provided the experience and understanding to comprehend how it is that others expect him to behave. While the behaviour in these instances may look the same, the reason for the actions may be slightly different, with the ADHD child knowing but not being able to carry out the expected behaviour and the looked after child not even knowing. Once again, this latter group of children might be able to tell you the rules, but it is sort of a rote recitation without really understanding what all of that means. For instance, they know you are not supposed to run in the hallway, but that does not count when you are scared of a noise you heard, or someone is chasing you, or when you are in a hurry to get to class.

The effects of abuse and neglect on the developing brain can result in academic learning difficulties as well as in emotional and mental health problems; however,

> When children enter school, there is a chance of recasting the die of early experience. The brain continues to grow and change. Even if the job has been partially bungled in the early years, much learning potential may be rescued. [Healy, 1990, p. 286]

The outcome for the particular individual depends upon what part of the brain has been damaged and, of course, the environment in which the brain has an opportunity, or not, to flourish. Sometimes there is pervasive developmental delay, and sometimes only certain parts of the brain are damaged. For example, a child may have motor problems, but otherwise be adequately competent cognitively. Many teachers and parents/carers will comment that the child certainly seems "clever enough" but will not apply himself to maths or to reading, or whatever it is that the child has trouble doing. Just because the brain is efficiently wired to do some things does not mean that it can do other things, too. In fact, no one has a perfect brain, and all of us have some form of learning weakness, but it may be that the weakness one person experiences is not so noticeable or dysfunctional as someone else's weakness. In our society, not being able to sew proficiently is much less detrimental than not being able to read, but, in reality, each is just a part of the brain working or not working with particular grace and acumen.

In summary, it can be see that both physical and emotional aspects of the brain can be affected by adverse conditions. Diminished growth in the left hemisphere of the brain leads to increased risk of depression; limbic system damage can affect emergence of panic disorders and post traumatic stress disorder; smaller growth in other parts of the brain can increase the risk of memory dysfunctions. Impairment in the connection between the two brain hemispheres has been linked to symptoms of attention deficit and hyperactivity. Many children who have been deprived of sensory stimulation suffer from sensory integration disorders, and children reared in environments that are negligent in the areas of affection and attention to needs often experience attachment disorders. Processing difficulties and perceptual dysfunctions, either visual or auditory, are not uncommon in both ADHD/ADD children and in adopted/looked after children.

Investigators are researching the plasticity of the brain because they are interested to learn more about the brain's ability to recover from severely compromised environments, from trauma and from other anomalies that may influence conduct and emotion. Brain scans and imaging have quite clearly indicated that, by three years of age, children who have been significantly abused and neglected have smaller brains than their peers who have had no such experiences (Glaser, 2000; Lehmann, 2002; Teicher, 2000). On the other hand, there is optimism in the research that suggests there is a fair amount of plasticity in the brain, and that the skills of damaged areas sometimes can be taken over by another part of the brain. Similarly, if a child did not have the necessary input at one point in his development, it is now thought that the information missed possibly may be acquired at a later date. This is certainly very encouraging information for parents, carers, and teachers who work with adopted/looked after children who have any one of many learning or living disabilities.

Neuro-imaging is looking at children's brains to see whether repeated exposure to trauma/terror changes the structure as well as the functioning of the brain, and, if so, how early this change takes place. Great advances have already been made in discovering how the brain works in the presence of traumatic stress. Since it is known that unregulated stress injures the brain, it is important for social workers, parents/carers, teachers, and therapists to figure out how children can be helped to develop stress regulation later in life if it were missed earlier on in the child's development (Huag-Storms, David, Dunn, & Bodenhauer-Davis, 2005).

In order for any of us to be truly helpful to ADHD/ADD adopted/looked after children, we need to make a concerted effort to walk in their shoes, to get inside their souls, to try to really understand how they feel and how they think. Just as they can recite rules without understanding them, we need to be careful that we do not mouth words without doing our best to know what the difficulties of these children feel like to them. It does not actually help us as adults to devise strategies for this group of children or to read lists of management techniques if we do not try to empathize with and appreciate the extent of the anxiety and frustration the children experience.

In this vein, instead of conceptualizing the "generic" child who is either ADHD/ADD or adopted/looked after, or both, it is important for adoptive parents, carers, and teachers to think specifically about the individual child. Your child may be like:

> *Andrew,* who is afraid to get up in the morning and go to school because he knows that he is going to muck up a whole bunch of things during his school day.
>
> *Charlotte,* who hates to go to PE because she knows how clumsy and awkward she is and she knows that the girls don't want her to be a part of their team.
>
> *Bruce,* who is scared of having his teacher shout at him for things he sometimes can do and sometimes can't do, but he never can predict just when he will get it right or wrong, and the shouting makes him too scared to do it right anyway.

If you are the parent/carer of one of these children, you know what it feels like for mums and dads, but if you are not, try to imagine how a mum feels because she is so used to getting phone calls from the school saying that her child is in trouble again that she does not even stay at home in the mornings so she will not be available when the school rings her.

Perhaps you are the teacher of an adopted/looked after child who brings emotional baggage and attentional difficulties to your classroom every day. You might be unsure if this child also has other specific learning disorders, but an assessment has not been arranged as yet. Even though you want to help the child to feel better and work more successfully in class, the specialists have not been available to teach you how to do this. Both you and the child will be treading water with neither of you knowing how to swim—a scary situation for each of you.

School, living in changing locations and feeling persistently out of control are situations that draw upon all of an adopted/looked after ADHD/ADD child's vulnerabilities. It would behove them and their parents/carers and teachers to contemplate their individual strengths and to introduce some aspects into their lives in which they can succeed. In his sensitive and brilliant work, Dr Robert Brooks stands out as a therapist and teacher who makes an enormous effort to understand the lives of complicated children. In *The Self Esteem Teacher* (1991), Brooks writes,

> I adopted the position that when children and adolescents become so-called disciplinary problems and when they rely on coping strategies that serve primarily to avoid challenges, our responsibility is to examine the ways in which our teaching or therapeutic style might be contributing to the use of these strategies. [p. 60]

Many practitioners have begun to think about altering a child's environment so as to enable the child to cope more effectively rather than always trying to change the child. It is through modifying the atmosphere and climate around the child that restructuring of the neural pathways can be helped; whereas demanding of the child behaviours and actions and thoughts that his/her brain is not programmed to handle will only produce increased frustration for everyone. Children in the care system are desperately in need of this kind of thinking, since their acquired coping skills do not often match up with what is being asked of them.

> Colin is nine years old and has been with his adoptive parents for four years. There are two other younger adopted children in this family and one older birth child. Colin confides that he always feels confused at home because everyone else seems to understand things that he doesn't. Somehow, he says, his shoes are never in the right place for being found or his books don't get from home to school. His father has promised him rewards that he never actually earns because he just doesn't see how he can do what his father wants him to do. The charts on the wall don't help because he forgets to look at them and there is too much on them anyway. Colin knows he is not supposed to hit his younger sister, but he doesn't know how else to keep her out of his room.

Children such as Colin not only have trouble at home, but they usually have considerable difficulty behaving and co-operating and understanding at school. ADHD / ADD adopted / looked after children who cannot cope with what is being asked of them in school are in need of a teaching style and a classroom environment that will enable them to focus and to learn in a more affirmative fashion.

Throughout your reading of this book, I hope very much that you will persistently keep in mind that Cinderella's glass slipper did not fit the feet of a lot of beautiful women, but when their mothers bought them shoes that did fit, they could dance as prettily as anyone else at the Ball.

CHAPTER THREE

The ADHD/ADD adopted/looked after child at home and in the community

"I want to make a new start but don't know where to begin. I wish things could have been done different, no matter how loud I talk, no one seems to listen." (Seventeen-year-old boy in care)

My father always told me that the best way to lose weight is to push yourself away from the table. That was, indeed, a good strategy as long as I did not then closet myself in my room with a box of chocolate biscuits. I point this out because it is my strong contention that there is no single strategy that works for everyone, and there are no absolute recipes that any of us can follow successfully to improve the behaviour and concentration of an ADHD child, of an adopted / looked after child or of any other child.

My own "recipe" for making things better is for each parent/ carer to try to know what makes his/her individual child tick. It is important to try to figure out when a child will go off the rails, will respond positively, will be able to succeed, and will quite definitely not be able to handle the situation. While this may be similar for some ADHD / ADD adopted / looked after children, the circumstances, especially for the adopted / looked after child, are so individualized and unique that generalities do not always apply. There is no magic formula.

When a child is removed from the birth family, various areas of psychosocial–emotional development can become disturbed. Attachment issues are very likely to surface. Children who have lost their birth mother are subject to maternal deprivation, even though the mother–child bond may not have been a healthy one. Environmental deprivation from an early age also makes the child vulnerable to a range of sensory deficits. These may include tactile defensiveness (not liking to touch or be touched or to walk on sand or grass or to play in messy materials, or other activities that involve the "touch" system). It may also include having sensory integration difficulties (not being able to make sense of the various stimuli coming into the brain and not being able to act correctly or appropriately to this stimuli), or to having proprioceptive weaknesses, not having an accurate or stable sense of your body in the space around you and not quite knowing/having a sense of where you are in relation to others or to things around you. A neglectful or abusive or poorly nutritioned milieu can result in one or many delays in physical, social, academic, emotional, and behavioural development.

A substantial body of research (Gunnar, 2001; Johnson, 2000), has shown that the consequences of early and severe deprivation can be rectified in some areas more readily than in others. For example, when children are put into good adoptive or foster care homes, physical growth, general intellectual performance, and language often improve. Other deficits are more recalcitrant, but not impossible to correct or ameliorate. For instance, young children who are under or poorly stimulated often are seen later to be those who have sensory processing difficulties. They are unable to take in, regulate, and respond to information in their environment.

It has been found among the Romanian cohort of adopted children that those enduring more than six months of institutional deprivation fared worse than those having shorter periods of inadequate or compromised experiences (Rutter, 1998). Infants and babies who have had a lack of opportunity to interact with others have been prevented from developing skills of self-regulation and social intercourse, so they may not learn how to play and work well with others in the future. As has been seen in the first two chapters, sensitive maternal deprivation can lead to abnormal brain development, poor internal regulation, behavioural difficulties, deficiencies in social interactions, and specific learning disorders.

Any or many of these deficits can become a worrying and difficult challenge with which the child and the parents/carers will need to contend. In order to respond effectively to whatever history the child is bringing into the home, two aspects must be considered:

- the experience and temperament of the child;
- the make-up and context of the family into which the child is being placed.

Not only should the parent/carer try to understand the particular child in question, but also, each parent/carer must work within the context of his/her own family. It is just not possible to try to make one size fit all. A normally quiet, laid-back, easy-going couple with a six-year-old birth daughter who plays happily on her own, loves her dolls, and causes no one any stress, might adopt a lively four-year-old boy who is energetic, cannot sit still for a minute, does not manage to focus on playing with any toy for more than a few seconds, and who has a temper like a time-bomb. This family is obviously going to require different adjustments from the family of five who all live whirlwind lives that depend upon high energy and less sedentary activities.

It is not to say that the second family is going to have it any easier (or harder) than the first family in the above instance; it is just to point out that the adjustments each family needs to make will vary. There is no right or wrong and no judgement in any of these situations, but if the dance does not work—and the larger the family, the harder it is to make all of the partnerships dance co-operatively—the more difficult the family (or school) situation will be. Just like parents and carers, teachers are each going to have chemistries that balance or upset certain student and classroom equations as well.

Although we all want magic wands and we look for quick solutions, parents and carers ultimately relax a little when they come to terms with the fact that there are no easy answers to these very problematic children. Sometimes we think we have hit upon a perfect solution because it works so well for a while, but then, discouragingly, the very wonderful strategy loses its effectiveness (that being the nature of growth and development, let alone of ADHD).

Even so, there is a certain freedom and acceptance and creativity in knowing and accepting the fact that there is not only one way of doing things because the family is no longer trying to meet someone else's expectations or criteria. Like everything else in life, there are ups and downs to living with all children. Living with ADHD/ADD adopted/looked after children probably carries one up more peaks and down more valleys than most families would travel, but that might bring moments of excitement and interest and serendipity that make life more enriching as well.

Despite the fact that we say there are no foolproof strategies or recipes, it is equally crucial to state that there are certain generalities that very often do apply to children with ADHD/ADD and frequently apply to adopted/looked after children as well. For example, it is quite unusual for any of these children not to do better in a home or a school that is structured, organized, and predictable than in one where chaos reigns. Both of these categories of children are at a loss to know how to internally regulate themselves, so monitoring and organizing their lives and schedules for them usually is a very helpful way of beginning to make a difference in their lives. If the child has already lived for months, or possibly for years, amid chaos and disorder, that child's brain will have made the necessary adjustments in its infrastructure to devise strategies that work for survival, but that same brain may not have family-living skills to cope with the new environment in which it is being asked to function. It will take patience and persistence on both the child's and the family's part to design a new neurological pattern.

While it is true that, short of absolute chaos, many perfectly well adjusted and successful children and adults actually do prefer a certain amount of spontaneity, disorder, and general mess in their lives, they are the ones who can create and find order internally in what may appear to others to be disorder. Creating order for themselves is not what ADHD children, or even ADHD adults, are able to do, so others need to do it for them. Most well functioning ADHD/ADD adults will tell you that they have marvellous secretaries or personal assistants, or amazingly organized and patient partners, or that they are totally dependent upon technology that organizes their lives for them.

Since most children who are in, or have come out of, the care system have little capacity to regulate their internal lives, creating a well arranged daily schedule is definitely an unrealistic expectation. Rather than expecting ADHD/ADD adopted/looked after children to tidy up their lives, it is more effective to have the adults provide a structure that becomes consistent and compatible for the child. It is important to create a very predictable environment for this group of children.

When the child is in a regulated family or classroom that is arranged so that the child can anticipate what will happen next and what will "happen if", it counteracts some of the stress and worry about this aspect of the situation and leaves the child with more energy to focus on the task at hand. It takes a long time, though, for some children to trust that the family or classroom will be stable and secure. Usually, they have to test this out quite a number of times—sometimes so often that the parent/carer/teacher gets exasperated and does not respond in the calm, desired, and predictable manner in which they would like to. Temporarily, this can seem to be a set-back for everyone involved, but life is not perfect, so telling the child (in a few short words) about why you or the child became derailed will be useful in helping all of you to get back on track.

Keeping the home as structured, consistent, and predictable as possible is a strategy that usually works in helping to mitigate unruly behaviour. It does not solve the problem, but it is a vital first step in designing a helpful environment. (See Tables 1 and 2.)

While it is true that most youngsters would thrive well in this sort of atmosphere, the adopted/looked after ADHD/ADD child actually requires an organized environment and a predictable schedule in order to function. When deviance from the usual plan must occur, preparing the child for the change is beneficial. What is difficult, and what differs so much for each child and family, tends to be how far in advance one tells the child about the anticipated change. For some, it is best to give about twenty-four hours' notice, so that the child has lots of time to think about it, talk about, even rehearse, how he/she might deal with the change. For other children, however, a day in advance may disrupt that whole day as well as the day of change. This child may do better being told at

Table 1. Structuring the environment to facilitate consistency and predictability

---

Physical aspects of the house:

The child's bedroom: his/her own bed and wardrobe/drawer/shelf space

Label drawers and shelves as to contents
Provide a few toys and books that child does not have to share with others
Hang up a short list of tidy-up chores: * make bed * pick clothes/toys off floor

Bathroom: child should have own toothbrush and towels and a place to put them

Study space: either in child's bedroom or in designated spot in the house

Space should have study tools appropriate to child's age.

If a child is a toddler or preschooler, it is still good to have a workspace with art materials available.

Play space: tell child where it is/is not all right to play, e.g., no toys in the lounge

Routines:

Waking, teeth brushing, washing, dressing should follow the same time and sequence each day. (This may differ at weekends.)

Meals need to be at same time every day.

Getting ready for school must have a plan: make packed lunch, collect back-pack, put homework, books, PE kit, musical instrument, etc. in pack. Parent to check.

Walking or driving to school is a good time to review the order of plans for that day. Reminder that child has karate after school or that the baby-sitter will be there when parents go out in the evening, etc.

After school: snack, homework, play time, bath—whatever order and schedule works for the whole family as well as the individual child, but it should be the same every day.

Bedtime: don't let it drag out and do the same every night: e.g., two stories, one song, one drink.

Table 2. What parents and carers can do to help.

- Be aware not to over-stimulate or over-exhaust.
- Limit the possibilities of distraction and diversion.
- Be predictable and consistent about all rules and routines, causes and consequences.
- Prepare the child for what will happen next and what will happen "if".
- Offer choices that are not yes or no: e.g., "Do you want cereal or eggs?"
- Allow for a certain flexibility within the structure: e.g., "You are sunburned today, so you may choose whether or not to have a bath."
- Write directions down (or draw pictures) as well as giving them orally.
  - Ask the child to repeat the instructions.
- Provide structure and plan programmes that help children to organize and monitor their own behaviour: "I'm going to read to you for three minutes. Turn the egg timer over and see if you can keep from talking until it is finished."
- Use pictures and manipulatives (objects child can touch/handle) when teaching new material or giving instructions.
- Play games and do exercises that practise desired behaviours (see Table 3 (p. 86) for ideas of how to help a child focus his attention).
- Choose one positive and one negative behaviour to work on each week.
  - Reward what is specifically well done, whether or not it was the behaviour "of the week".
  - Contain negative behaviour but don't "punish" all of it all of the time.

breakfast time that there will be a supply teacher in class that morning, or that grandma, not mum, will be home after school to make the child's dinner. Knowing your child well will help to guide you in making decisions about how much advance preparation your particular child requires.

Almost categorically, "surprises" and absolutely last-minute alterations of plans do not work well for adopted/looked after ADHD/ADD children. For example, it would be a real mistake to plan a surprise party for this child. We already know that most adopted/looked after ADHD/ADD children do poorly when they are caught off-guard and are unprepared, so knowingly putting these children in a new or startling situation is bringing on a disruption that could, and should, be avoided. Surprises to these children are synonymous with chaos, and one can expect that the child will not be able to cope. Moreover, surprises upset one's internal balance. If setting oneself straight is not something a child is good at, catching the child unaware most likely will be something the parent/carer/teacher will want to avoid.

The most successful birthday parties for this group of children, incidentally, are the small ones. If your child has managed to make just one or two friends, this is the time to be grateful, and do not invite the whole neighbourhood or the whole class to make up for what may seem to you like too few friends. While some children might be happiest staying at home with one or two friends, others will find it too hard to share their toys and their personal space. These children will like going to a park, to the cinema, to a football game, to the science museum, or to some other place where each child can be expected to take in the activity in a way that suits him/her most comfortably. Again, finding an activity that your child enjoys and does reasonably well is the best place to start.

Another generality that leads to strategic planning for the adopted/looked after ADHD/ADD child both at home and at school pertains to competition. Most youngsters in either or both of these categories fall apart in competitive situations. They are too used to losing, so will do everything they possibly can to disrupt any activity that speaks of winners and losers. Here enters the class clown the minute the teacher announces a spelling test, or a prize for the student who learns the multiplication tables first, or even a chance to be first in the queue at break-time for the child whose desk top is the cleanest. Children need to be settled and confident and have a certain amount of self-esteem before they can pit themselves against others. Children with ADHD/ADD and/or children who have been in the care system project a certain "face" about losing, but they do not actually have the self-confidence they need to handle losing. It is more beneficial just to let them try to improve in whatever the task is rather than having them work to do it better than someone else.

It is important to think about temperament when devising strategies that will work for the child in your care—and for you!

When there is a clash between temperament and environment, volcanic eruption can be the outcome. Successful strategies are those that find a link between the child and the surroundings—not those that require the child to meet the needs of the environment. Exuberant, boisterous children are just as hard to calm down as shy, quiet children are to light up, but thinking very specifically about what each child responds to, and requires in order to respond, is a better plan than insisting upon someone else's design that does not fit your child. Moreover, if the adult in charge keeps attempting to squeeze the square peg into the round hole, it will only make everyone feel uncomfortable and annoyed, resulting in double trouble.

Children sometimes have the best answers to the problem. If a certain task needs to be done and nothing you are trying or have tried works, it might be worth asking the child.

"Jason, I get the message that you don't like doing maths homework, but we actually have no choice about this, so I need your help. According to your teacher, my job is to look at your completed maths page and sign off that you did the work. Your job is to do the ten problems. Do you have an idea of how we are going to accomplish this task tonight?"

Asking Jason gives him a chance to take responsibility, to problem solve, to do something his own way. If he cannot come up with a solution, you can remind him that until he is able to take control of himself, you will be there to do it for him.

If accomplishing homework continuously presents tantrums and difficulties at home, I would suggest that the parent/carer takes the control in a slightly altered sense. The teacher will not be thrilled about this, and the reader may not be either, but in this situation, as a parent, I wouldn't struggle over all ten problems. I would point out to Jason that you are willing for him to do five problems and you will sign the homework, saying it was the best that both you and he could do. Then, let him pay the consequences at school. This in itself might motivate him to do all ten, or it may not, but at least it could avoid major catastrophe at home and it is a step in the right direction. One will hope that the teacher thinks so too. A subsequent conversation between parent and teacher will be useful.

Generally speaking, many adopted/looked after ADHD/ADD children tend not to have brilliant social skills. The strategies that usually work in these instances involve talking about "the obvious", which is not always so obvious to them. Adults need to talk about and explain things that normally would not need explaining. This can be particularly true for children who have specific learning disorders along with their ADHD/ADD. It is quite common to hear these children say, "Nobody ever told me that." In fact, they are right. Nobody ever told them because nobody ever would have thought that they had to do so. What other children get by osmosis, this group of children seems oblivious to. Children who do not have good social skills do not "get" the idea of what everyone else just internalizes. Most toddlers will often sit or stand for quite a long time, virtually staring at older children. They are absorbing all kinds of information when they do this. It is how they learn about social interactions. By the time these children get to school, they will have some idea of how other children play together. Little ones who have never been taken to the park, the beach, outside in a neighbourhood, even to a shopping centre will not have had the opportunity to make these observations and to integrate them into their social thinking.

Seven-year-olds watching other children in the playground will intuitively appreciate that most of the time it is best to wait your turn, although you would much rather not. They learn that sharing is the done thing, despite the fact that they would like to keep the ball all to themselves. They accept the idea of saying "Sorry", even if they are not, because they realize that it keeps you out of trouble or makes you more friends. Since these children are relatively in charge of their inner controls, they are able to turn down the impulse buttons and to organize a bit of patience and empathy. Unfortunately, it is beyond the power of many adopted/looked after children and most ADHD children to regulate these control systems, or even to recognize that they need to do so.

Strategies that are useful for dealing with social skills again vary according to each child, but I have found looking at pictures of children playing, and talking with a child about these pictures can help. "What do you think is happening in this photo? What are the children doing? Do you think everyone is having a good time? What do you suppose this child without a sand spade is feeling? Is there a leader in this group? If you were in this photo, where would you like to be in it?" Video can be good for this too—sometimes without the sound first time around. Try to involve the child in seeing different points of view and in empathizing with various children in the pictures. Teachers can do this in small groups in classrooms just as easily as parents/carers can do it in the home. The adult might ask children to write bubble words or phrases above each person in the picture to express what that person is thinking or feeling.

It is also good to rehearse situations before they happen. If a friend has been invited for a play afternoon, it can be useful to ask Samantha if she would like to put some toys away because they are too hard to share with others, or to talk about what she would like to do with her friend. Again, a short afternoon with much structure is a good starter. The adult need not be ever-present, but should be pretty close at hand for supportive intervention.

The adopted/looked after ADHD/ADD child at home

> For Daniel, life at home meant a lot of hiding and fighting and being tough and not caring. It meant being hungry and stealing things for mother and making sure you knew where your sister was. It meant not accepting "gifts" because you always have to pay for them somehow, or else you just get to like them and they go back to the store anyway. Life at home came with getting smacked even though you didn't know why or not getting smacked when you thought you might. At night, you stayed awake a lot to make sure your sister didn't scream.

> Life at home for Christie meant finding food for you and your little brother and not telling your mother where you got it. It meant being quiet and not being noticed but paying attention to where that boyfriend has got to, and being sure you put the groceries away when there were any so you know what you could take out and hide under your bed. Home was shutting up and not needing anything from anyone. It was watching and watching but not letting anyone see you.

It is already clear that the adopted/looked after child who is also ADHD/ADD is not an easy child with whom to live at home, and, as has been previously alluded to, even parents and carers who have considered themselves to be quite calm and organized individuals, find that they become more tense, uptight, stressed, somewhat chaotic care-givers when living with the combination of

ADHD / ADD and adoption or being looked after. Unfortunately, by the time they receive professional help, the parents / carers are usually in such a state themselves that the therapist often focuses on the adult behaviour, seeing it as cause for the child's dysfunction. Families seeking professional input for adopted / looked after ADHD / ADD children must be very sure that they go to a therapist who has a good working knowledge and some experience with the kinds of issues these children can bring into a family. Although there are many different kinds of therapeutic approaches, most of which can be equally beneficial, a therapist who is well versed in the issues of both adoption / being in care and of attention disorders should be the highest priority when choosing a professional and mode of intervention.

> ... Those moods affected the atmosphere of the entire house. I remember I wanted to slap him ... Occasionally I actually did hit him. ... It wasn't me, the woman who suddenly leapt out of me at those moments ... One moment the hatred, the next the love ... I didn't know I had it in me. [Kay, 1998, p. 153]

Although ADHD / ADD children who are born into stable, loving families will have been exposed to appropriate stimulation and will have had environments that promote learning readiness, they may not have been able to utilize all that has been positive in their environment. While parental patience is probably wearing thin after several years of living with an ADHD / ADD child, at least this child carries somewhat lighter baggage than the child who has spent weeks, months, years experiencing abuse and neglect in addition to attention problems.

The looked after or adopted baby who enters the world with a genetic background of attention difficulties may have inadvertently provoked worse treatment for himself in a fragile home environment than the non-ADHD child would have done, because the behaviour and emotional state of ADHD / ADD children tends to be more volatile and harder to regulate or to manage than the non-ADHD child's. An infant with a quiet temperament and with a certain resiliency sometimes is less likely to become the scapegoated or afflicted child in a violent home. Children with ADHD, however, make themselves known through their need and demand for attention and because of their own explosive natures. These children are at greater risk for being abused and are less likely to receive positive attention and affection when they live in unsettled and/or hostile settings. Their impulsivity easily attracts the wrath of those who are in charge of their care.

> Ian says, "I have a lot of problems because I just get angry so easily. I don't know why that is, but I do. I can't stop myself when it happens, and then I get in trouble."

Thus, the infant who has a genetic inheritance of ADHD/ADD will stand a better chance in a home setting that can understand and meet the needs of a baby who is poor at self-regulation, whose schedule is erratic, and whose temperament fluctuates. For the neurological and self-protective reasons talked about earlier, if a baby who has no genetic background for ADHD/ADD is brought up in an environment of limited or negative stimulation, of abuse, neglect, violence, and disorganization, this child may well begin to take on the characteristics of an ADHD/ADD child. Children who are not provided with appropriate stimulation sometimes begin to create their own (milder) forms of autistic-like behaviour, where they might twirl, or make noises, or move about continuously so as to bring some interest into their environment. Alternatively, of course, they might just vegetate and "check out". The same is true if there is too much stimulation: an overloaded infant is likely either to go into shut-down mode or to over-respond to everything. It is not surprising, then, that many children who are adopted/looked after but who have no genetic propensity to have acquired ADHD/ADD, nevertheless appear to have problems with attention when they enter their new families or homes.

A young infant's attention is enhanced when there is a strong attachment between child and care-taker. When the baby is held, fed, bathed, and played with, the primary care-taker seeks to make a connection with the baby's eyes. The baby and care-taker focus on one another, mimicking one another's expressions and sounds. If a baby does not have these kinds of experiences on a regular basis, both the attachment and the ability to attend will be diminished. Parents typically invest a lot of time and energy in connecting with their infant, which is what helps to promote the infant's social–emotional development as well as his/her cognition and attention.

Although ADHD / ADD infants in any home will have more trouble engaging with their care-takers than do other infants, they will be especially jeopardized if they are never even asked to engage, or if their lack of engagement is perceived by the care-taker as rejection.

Although intelligence in and of itself is not the specific issue at hand concerning most children with attention difficulties, it is not unusual for the ADHD / ADD adopted / looked after child to have specific learning and living dysfunctions. Living in the context of a new family—or several sequential families—is a complicated task for any child. This alone may be a job that is too overwhelming for most children. For the child in care who also has attention problems, just figuring out how to get through a day at home will be enormously stressful. As consistency has not been a part of their lives in the past, they have little or no expectation of daily routines and scheduled lives. They do not have a concept of predictability, so are likely not to understand "what happens next", and are very poor at grasping the idea of cause and consequence. We already know that they are internally fragile children, but, because they have trouble controlling their moods and behaviours, and because no one has ever helped them with this in the past, they may well see their behaviour as being perfectly normal. In fact, because the outside world has already taught children in the care system that adults cannot be trusted and that change happens suddenly and irrationally no matter what the child does, they could be forgiven for assuming that this is what life is all about. Therefore, the fact that they cannot meet the "demands" of the new family must be very confusing and discouraging to them. Clearly, children in this situation require an enormous amount of help, understanding, patience, and endurance.

It is quite common among adopted / looked after and ADHD / ADD children that they do not (will not or cannot) take responsibility for their own behaviour. Sometimes it is hard to figure out if they really do not appreciate that they are responsible for whatever happened or if they are protectively covering up. Some of this is, developmentally, a two-year-old stage of thinking and behaving: i.e., the milk could not possibly have spilled itself, but that is what the six- or eight-year-old child insists has happened. While one expects this at age two, it is not something one likes to see in the eight-, nine-, and ten-year-old.

When the consequences of misbehaviour, as in the relatively minor case above, were previously very drastic, one can appreciate why the child in care may have begun to convince himself that he/she is not responsible for what has happened. In situations where the child was severely punished for quite innocuous misdemeanours, or the child never knew if the behaviour would produce a positive or negative response, the connection between cause and consequence would have been difficult to formulate. It is always best for a child to begin learning quite young that "If I do this, then that will happen". The "this" and the "that" can be either positive or negative, as in, "If I play with my food and throw it on the floor, mummy will take it away from me", or, "If I pick up all my toys, mummy will read me an extra story". Sadly, such benign situations do not happen in dysfunctional families. Moreover, children in care with attention disorders often miss out on this cause and consequence sequence because they may have been distracted by something else (often fear) that interrupted their thinking process during the sequence. These are frequently the children who say things like, "I didn't do anything wrong, but the teacher always punishes me for whatever happens."

In his/her own mind, this same child is never at fault for anything. It is always someone else who was wrong or who is to be blamed or who is the cause of the problem. In the mind of the child who cannot take responsibility for his behaviour, all streets are one-way, and the child has determined that he is the one going in the right direction. In fact, from his own working model, it *is* the safest way to travel, because this child has already convinced himself that taking responsibility inevitably means trouble. Sometimes trouble comes anyway (like getting a beating), but if you "didn't do it", then you can more easily disassociate yourself from the beating—with the end result that there is no meaning to cause and consequence. Teaching the well-defended child to learn about his own behaviour can be quite an arduous task and needs to begin in a very positive mode—not with what you did wrong, but what you did right! Rewards are powerful in these situations, and can be used often for reinforcing positive behaviour.

When beginning the process of teaching a child about assuming responsibility for his/her own actions and deeds, it is well to look at the developmental level of the child who comes into the home.

Although the child may be six years of age, and may even act six or older in some street-wise or other ways, emotionally and neurologically the child may well be functioning at a much younger level. Perhaps the child is not actually mature enough to take responsibility for her behaviour, or emotionally the child may not be ready to cope with that much responsibility. If a child persists in blaming others, it is a sign to the parents/carers or teachers that the child is not ready to assume responsibility for his behaviour and that the adult should therefore stay in charge for a while longer. It is likely that this will be very uneven development, so that in some aspects of the child's life the child may be perfectly capable of managing, while in other areas he may still require a lot of external input. Much of this depends upon the neurological sophistication of that individual child and of what happened earlier in her experiences.

In the house that Jack built

We often talk about children in care not having a firm foundation upon which to build a strong future. It is true that we all know a building cannot stand on a weak foundation. The irony for the adopted child is that they already have, for several years, been constructing their house. Now they find that trying to build a foundation when there is already a house on top is not an easy job either. Parents and carers have a very laborious challenge as they struggle with their children to put one solid brick on top of another while remoulding a stronger and more durable base at the same time.

Children with ADHD/ADD are not the best construction engineers either. They may have good ideas and artistically clever designs, but carrying out the building of these schemata is tricky for them. Over the years, I have worked with many very intelligent ADHD/ADD children who have a project in mind that is actually probably too hard for anyone, let alone someone with attention difficulties, to construct. When it does not work, they become increasingly frustrated and angry. Even with adult scaffolding to support both their project and their emotions, these children can fly way out of control over what seems to others like a fairly minor incident.

Erica is eight years old. She is a good artist and likes to do arts and crafts projects although her difficulties with attention frequently get in her way with completing them. In trying to build a bridge with lolly-sticks, Erica finds that she has a design in her head that is just not working when she tries to construct it. Like most children, she becomes annoyed and discouraged, but, unlike most children, she is not able to give it a smash or two or cry a bit or call it stupid names. Erica has taken this "defeat" to extraordinary proportions and tries to smash everyone else's project as well as her own. Screaming, fighting, hurling abuse at anyone who tries to talk to her, she finally dashes out of the room—an action that proved to be safer for her and everyone else.

As a child who has had seventeen different home placements and who has a very short attention span, Erica has seen this failed project as one more downward spiral: "I never can do anything; I'm so stupid; the teacher wouldn't help me; nobody likes me," and so forth.

Although at the time of the explosion it is hard for anyone around the Ericas of the world to be calm and rational, we do need to think about these kinds of children so that we can protect them from themselves as well as from others who get in the way of their wrath. Erica's life has not given her much reason to be able to focus on and complete a task or to take control of things she has in mind to do. Her life of interruption and sadness has rightfully contributed to her self-defeating attitude, and any efforts she may have made in the past to assume some responsibility or control of her inner self probably came to little fruition. Erica operates at quite an early, almost primitive, level of emotional and psychological development because she has no alternative skills that work.

In general, neither ADHD / ADD nor adopted / looked after children spend much time focusing on the task at hand, unless it is a task of especially high interest, and then they are likely to focus so intently that there is no budging them. This does not make for a very malleable individual with whom to live. It also can be quite a shock for the parent / carer who is not familiar with this kind of behaviour. Mostly, it is quite confusing when, ninety per cent of the time, the child does not attend to anything for more than a few minutes, but then sits at the computer or in front of the television for hours on end. Interestingly, these are also children who sometimes can, unlike Erica, work at a project very intensely (if no one gets in their way and it is going well).

Without input and support, the parent/carer probably is not able to devise an emotional or a literal plan of action to cope with the particular characteristics and actions of these special needs children. Even very good and experienced parents need more professional insight and training when asked to take on ADHD/ADD children as adopted or looked after new people in their household. Since they are not youngsters who respond to "normal" parenting, different plans must be put in place in order to meet the needs of children who do not, will not, cannot respond as most other children do. Knowing more about ADHD/ADD and about the issues adopted and looked after children often present certainly does not solve all of the difficulties, but it does go a long way in helping to mitigate some of the frustration on both sides. When parents, carers, and teachers understand better about why a child might be acting and feeling and thinking the way he/she does, it does make the adult act, feel, and think differently too.

Some behaviours that ADHD/ADD adopted/looked after children might exhibit

Typically, both ADHD/ADD and adopted/looked after children have trouble following relatively simple directions; they do not obey house-rules; they have incredibly messy rooms in which they never can find anything they might need. Those with hyperactivity are often loud and boisterous to the extreme; they move from one toy to another before even looking at the first toy; they are never satisfied with or gratified by anything anyone offers or anything they do themselves. They do not remember to do their household chores, or, if they do remember, they probably do them carelessly or incompletely. Adults in charge of these children will typically use many of the same adjectives to describe the child: whirlwind, hyper, non-stop, exhausting, uncontrollable . . .

Children without hyperactivity are less noisy and obstreperous, but they are equally frustrating because they too cannot amuse themselves and they find it hard to make, or follow through with, a plan of action. Like their ADHD cohorts, they forget things, lose things, struggle to make friends or keep friends, and are rarely satisfied with the food, toys, activities, and entertainment that are offered to them.

Similar to ADHD children, those without hyperactivity do not excel at efficiency. Moreover, they find it impossible to meet the expectations that people have of other children of the same age.

The unpredictable and erratic moods of adopted/looked after ADHD/ADD children make them difficult for parents and carers both at home and in the community. These are not children one wants to take to the supermarket, out to a restaurant, on a holiday, or even to grandma's house—maybe especially to grandma's house—as most friends and family are quick to blame the parents of these children for their unmanageable behaviour. Moodiness can take the form of shutting down/shutting out so that the child is non-compliant and vapid. Alternatively, the moodiness can fall anywhere along a continuum of emotions, culminating in the explosive rages that often characterize looked after, adopted, and ADHD children.

It must be remembered that neither being adopted/looked after nor being ADHD/ADD is necessarily fun or easy for the child either. While most adopted children actually are pleased to be in a safe and happy family, they still bring a history with them that is different from other children and that might get in their way frequently or from time to time. No matter how kind and loving the new family is, the past cannot be erased or forgotten, and twinges of what happened to them in an earlier life may assault them at any time—almost always without warning. A smell, seeing someone in the shopping centre who looks like someone they knew, a birthday—just about anything can evoke a memory, some good, many not so happy.

Children who are looked after are rarely grateful for their situation. While they may feel safer and better fed and cared for, they suffer from not being adopted, which, in the cruelty of children's bullying and in the school playground, is a "higher status" category than being looked after. Despite the fact that many of these children do better in long-term foster care than they might do elsewhere, and despite what carers and professionals do to support this view, the general mode of other children and society at large deems it better to be adopted. Therefore, the lives of these children are complicated, even before the element of ADHD/ADD walks through the door. Most of these children recognize that they are not doing what other children their age do, a fact that can make them both sad and defiant. They may observe that other children understand things or follow through on tasks or have more friends than they do, even though they usually do not know why this is true.

Children with ADHD/ADD often feel bad about themselves and know they are different, but they do not really understand why. Children in this situation tell us that they wish they could be like everyone else, but they do not know how to be. When adults say things like "be more patient", "wait your turn", "don't grab things from your brother", or "settle down", ADHD/ADD children have little or no capacity to mobilize or maintain that behaviour. They are unable to internalize what it feels like to live that way or to behave that way consistently. Moreover, it is extremely tiring for them to act in a manner that is virtually alien to their nature, so if they manage to do what they are supposed to for a short while, they are probably completely exhausted subsequently, which is one reason why they come home from school and fall apart.

The truth is, none of us is good at maintaining behaviour that is uncomfortable or strange to us. People go off diets because dieting is difficult behaviour to sustain day after day. People learning foreign languages find it exhausting to try to speak and listen all day to the new language. As a result, all of us retreat from the behaviours we would like to stick with because it is too hard to persist with them. This is what the ADHD/ADD and the adopted/looked after children do, too. They may try for a while, but then they run out of steam and they fall back on to what comes more naturally for them. Parents and teachers will say "they can do it if they try", and that may be true, but it is very short-lived. More often than not, the children do try and do want to do things differently, but they simply cannot keep up whatever it is they are being required to do.

Managing your ADHD/ADD adopted/looked after child at home can be one of the most difficult tasks of all because of the fact that some ADHD/adopted and looked after children can hold themselves together for a short time while they are out, or sometimes even while they are at school, and then they collapse when they arrive home. In essence, this should be very flattering, because it means they feel safe and secure at home; however, in reality, one might sometimes wish they did not feel quite that content so they would behave reasonably. It is, of course, the ultimate paradox, because, as a parent/carer, one does everything possible to make a child feel comfortable, understood, accepted—and then, in this case, the reward one reaps is utter disaster. Usually, there is no point in talking this over with the child because it is not very likely to change things. The child may understand, but cannot change. Talking on and on about it may just make him/her feel worse.

On a more cheerful note, while there is much that is hard to manage, difficult to understand, annoying and hurtful to live with, there are also many bright sides to children with attention difficulties. Childhood is the most problematic period in the life stages of someone with ADHD. Often, as adults, they are witty, clever, innovative, highly accomplished individuals, even though most people do not outgrow having an attention deficit, which is generally seen as being a life-long disorder. It is the management of the disorder that can be altered. When allowed the freedom to choose their own job or occupation and to use their unique style to their distinct advantage, many ADHD adults are tremendously successful in their professions and can be the life and soul of a party. Many are fun, fast, full of vibrancy and valour. Granted, they usually need a gifted and patient secretary or personal assistant or partner, but there is no reason to despair about a significant number of ADHD/adopted adults if concomitant emotional and psychological difficulties are adequately addressed and remediated. (See Appendix II, which presents several examples of adults who are still struggling with ADHD/ADD issues, but who are functioning relatively well in many aspects of their lives.)

The plan of action

ADHD children almost never plan or plot their behaviour. They do not lie in bed in the morning organizing strategies for disrupting everyone's day. If they were this successful at planning, they would not be ADHD! However, adopted/looked after children may indeed try to "plot" their behaviour, because they have been used to doing so in self-defence. Since they tend not to trust adults and to be angrier than other children, they may think about vindication and retaliation, and/or they may have more of a self-preservation strategy of "I'll get you before you can get me."

For those adopted/looked after children who are also ADHD, the "plan" probably does not very often materialize because they are not organized enough to carry it through and because their impulsive nature will waylay whatever plan they thought to enact anyway, but these digressions do not mitigate the intention. These children have the potential to become less manageable, less rational, more disruptive, and more violent than their non-adopted/looked after ADHD peers because they have even more anger, hurt, and frustration rumbling around inside of them. They also will trust less the adults who are trying to help them. As with everything else, though, there probably are many adopted and looked after children who wake up in the morning trying to work out how they can be really "good" all day without getting into any trouble.

Like all other children, the vast majority of adopted/looked after ADHD/ADD children want to do the right thing; they just cannot manage to do it. They are so easily distracted that they forget the strategies they have been taught that would make things better for themselves and others. Usually, these children have learned intellectually what would be the proper way to behave—they can give you all of the right answers—but what they have not learned is how to control their impulsive responses.

> Nathan is seven and a half years old, an extremely clever lad, adopted at four years of age. He has the prototypical background of neglect and malnutrition that is seen in so many adopted children and the stereotypical behaviours of numerous ADHD boys. Following a morning of non-stop confrontation with another boy his age, George, who is also adopted and ADHD, Nathan, George and I talk about their behaviour. As I was not with the boys in the morning, I had the advantage of being able to ask some "naïve" and useful questions.
>
> "So, Nat, tell me a little about what happened this morning."
>
> Nathan: "Well, George was really bothering me a lot and I know I should have ignored him, but I just couldn't do it. Besides, he kept following me and bugging me, so I had to hit him."
>
> I asked George what he thought about this.
>
> George: "Yeah, well I guess I was being too aggressive [yes, his word!], and I know I should have stopped, but I couldn't. I really don't know why I kept bugging him. Something inside me. I'm sorry now, but I wasn't then."

I asked if Nathan was sorry.

Nathan: "I was just really angry so I couldn't do anything right. It was his fault, but I didn't make it better."

The level of awareness in both of these boys was somewhat startling to me, and emphasizes how often ADHD children do really know what is going on and do really want to behave better. While I talked to the boys, we were all sitting on the floor, the boys about six feet apart, each playing with his own sand tray. They were relaxed, engaged in their play, and thus able to talk about the situation, but, discouragingly, neither of the boys felt that he was capable of doing things differently next time. Nathan said: "I never can control myself at the time. Later, I wish that I had."

What does all of this tell us? What can we learn from the children who are trying to let us know what happens to them and how they feel about it?

This is another chance to review altering the child's environment to meet the child's needs. The youngster who is physically disabled has a huge advantage in this respect because we do not ask that child to do what he/she cannot do. We make it possible for the child to do it, or we do it for the child. Similarly, we do not expect toddlers to do what school children can do; we take the necessary equipment or provide the safety net for the toddler in order to accommodate that child's needs. The ADHD/ADD adopted/looked after child must be given this opportunity as well.

It is hard when a child is chronologically one age and emotionally another, but that is not the child's fault. Steps toward advancement come slowly, and only with a lot of scaffolding. If Nathan says "I never can control myself at the time", then it is up to the adults in Nathan's environment either to provide the controls he has not yet learned, or to avoid putting him in the stressful situation until he has acquired the skills he needs in order to manage his own behaviour.

Choices and self control

ADHD/ADD adopted/looked after children are accustomed to feeling out of control. Their minds are not in synchrony with their bodies, which is why they know the school rules, but very rarely carry them out, and why their impulses usually win the race between thinking and doing. As adults, we have an important role to play in the child's life in teaching the child self-control, remembering that this is not going to come easily to the child in question. Learning to make choices and learning how to follow through on a choice is one way of gaining self-control. A particularly good choice for an ADHD child to learn how to make is one of building in break-times. The child will like learning about taking a planned time-off, so this is often an excellent place to start. All of us are more inclined to learn something if it seems fun or rewarding or worth learning. We tend to shy away from learning things that seem too hard or a waste of time. ADHD and children in care respond well to rewards that they are in charge of, and taking a break can easily be one of these. Children with an attention deficit need many more than the usual number of rest periods, although the "rest" may be very active. For many people, these constant interruptions would interfere with the flow of what is being taught or learned, but having trouble with paying attention is often rectified by frequent short stretches between innings. The important aspect of this plan is that the child must learn that concentration improves with *planned* breaks, not with random breaks.

This is one example of how it works.

> Marsha, I see you have some writing work to do for school tonight. What I want you to do is write three sentences, and then take a break by coming down to the kitchen to see me. Maybe you could read me your three sentences when you come, but you don't have to. I'll give you a . . . (star on the chart, glass of juice, hug, etc.) when you come to see me. Then you go back upstairs and write another three sentences. It is good for you to take breaks when you work because it helps you to . . . (do your work better, focus on your work, feel better, get some exercise, etc.).

The above scenario is only one example, and it is why you must know your child well. Some people will read this and feel that it would never work for them, but perhaps some version of this scenario could work, like having the child in the same room as you so that you can be sure the three sentences (or might it be just one sentence?) gets written. Maybe you need to ask the child how many sentences should be written before the break period comes in, or maybe the child needs to work with a five-minute timer. Maybe you *do* need to see or hear the sentences to be sure the child has actually written them. Different strategies work with each individual child and family, but the overall idea of teaching the child a strategy that will work for him is the way forward to helping you manage the child and the child to managing him/herself.

Rewards/reinforcers

Behaviour management can hardly be mentioned today without a discussion about the concomitant star-charts that are generally associated with behavioural therapy. Behaviour modification comprises rewards and punishments, but rewards are often a controversial topic because many people believe that one should not reward a child for behaviour that is expected. If we look at infancy, a baby smiles at us, and we almost automatically smile back. That is the infant's reward, and so she does it again, and so do we. We do expect that infants will smile, but we go on rewarding them for a very long time in their smile-learning process. They are not one-trial learners, but eventually, smiling brings its own rewards to the child (and to the adult!), and it becomes a spontaneous activity, executed only at appropriate times because we do not smile at the baby who has done something naughty. Many of us will have experienced the cheeky smile of a toddler who thinks that his naughty behaviour will go unnoticed if he puts on his cute little smile for us. It is a clearer message if we do not let him get away with this and if we only reward behaviours we want to reinforce.

Even as adults, we do things that bring us rewards. We go to jobs for pay cheques; we work so that we can afford holidays; we eat well or exercise so that we can feel healthy; we make friends so that we can have support and understanding and be with others socially; we practise instruments for the joy of playing music. We also do some things we do not like doing or that we have to do because the consequence of not doing them (the punishment) is worse than the act of doing them, i.e., we would get sacked from a job if we did not show up on time; we would get a ticket if we broke the speed limit; we might get bugs and rats in the house if we did not do a bit of housecleaning.

Like everyone else, ADHD/ADD children also work for rewards, but frequently the value of the reward dies quickly, almost before two stars can hit the chart. On the other hand, the adopted/looked after children may sometimes work to avoid the reward because the fear of failure is too great. These children will sabotage the reward system before it can even start. If you sense that your child or student falls into this category, you will need to change the incentive to meet the child's needs or temperament. It is important, therefore, to constantly re-evaluate the actual reinforcement value of any given reward. A nod of approval may be enough of an early reward for a child who has been unable to accept reinforcement of positive behaviour.

> Cassie is just over three years old and was adopted ten months ago. Her mother said they had recently begun a star chart for her on which she gets stars each time her mother doesn't have to say "No" to her at the dinner table. Cassie seemed to be earning very few stars, so she and her mother were both feeling unhappy about it.
>
> I suggested that she might reward Cassie instead for everything she did well at the dinner table. If she said "Please" or if she made an attempt to eat her food, or if she smiled at her sister, she could get a star for any or all of those positive behaviours.

Enhancing the amount of positive feelings between parent and child is an important first step in creating attachment and the incentive to do better. Being with a child while the child plays (allowing the child to direct the activity rather than the adult leading it), doing something together that both parent/carer and child enjoy, no matter how short a time it lasts, and providing reinforcement for the positive behaviours you want to see more of all enable the frequency of desired behaviour to increase. Noticing and commenting on positive behaviours at least twice a day could become the goal of the parent/carer/teacher. Their own reinforcement in doing so will be improved attitude and compliance from the child.

In general, children with concentration problems need more positive and negative consequences for longer periods of time than children without attention difficulties. Children in the care system, however, can be more complex *vis-à-vis* rewards because their early experiences may have provided them with a script that is contrary to the way the programme is supposed to read. Children with sexual abuse in their background may have been given sweets and treats in exchange for giving their bodies. Children with substance-addicted parents may have been promised a piece of the profit if they went out to steal products or money for the parent. Ultimately, they may or may not have been given their share of the profit. Often, they learnt to swipe their own percentage off the top before handing over the remainder. One has to be very careful about rewards with children in the care system, anticipating that some of these children will be wary or untrusting of the promised gift.

Rewards do not need to be tangible, and it may be that a quick word of praise is more effective for some adopted/looked after ADHD/ADD children. "Nice work, Holly," can be very gratifying to a child who is not yet ready to accept any other reward or even greater verbal praise. Many teachers and parents have experienced the child who will immediately tear up her work after having received just the tiniest bit of praise for it. Often with children who have learning disorders or attention problems, they do not trust that they will ever be able to succeed again, so they do not want that "good" piece of work held up as an example of "what you can do when you try". This happens both at home and at school. In these instances, it might be more effective simply to give that child a bit of attention by asking the child to tell you about what she drew, or by asking the child who brings a picture home from school if she wants you to put it on the refrigerator or not. It might be best not to say anything about its being a pretty picture or a good drawing or anything else that can imply judgement.

Some of the most effective reinforcements, indeed, are not those that are tangible or that cost money. Many children like being able to earn a later bedtime on weekends, a day out with a parent/carer, a day off from doing household chores, a chance to not have to do homework one evening. Some children would like to sleep out of doors in a tent; others would like to choose what they eat for dinner one night a week; some would rather not have to brush their teeth before going to bed; some would like to have a bag of biscuits in their room. While it is not always possible to comply with these requests, most are all right once in a while. Not brushing your teeth every night is a bad thing, but not brushing them one night a week (particularly if it is in exchange for not arguing at the dinner table) is not really going to make too much difference. Since most ADHD/

ADD children and many adopted/looked after children are short on durability, it is unlikely that the reward is going to persist for very long anyway, so it is often safe to assume that "this too will pass". Whatever it was that the child wanted so intensely last week will probably be dropped in favour of something else next week.

Usually, children will tell you exactly what they would like, although often their choices are not at all reasonable or within the realm of possibility. Even so, it gives you an idea of what appeals to them, and you may be able to come to some sort of compromise. Sometimes the child just chooses an outrageous reinforcement to test you. They do not necessarily want what they chose, but they do want to see if you will give it to them.

In the learning process of gaining self-control, it is best to try to involve the child in the planning of when and how a reward system will work. It should be very small and very specific. "Good behaviour", for example, has absolutely no meaning at all. What one person considers good might be very different from another person's idea of good. The expected behaviour must be spelled out, and it must involve the child's input. It is important for the success of these projects to hear what the child needs and wants, too.

If mum wants Kurt to tidy up his room, she needs to tell Kurt what that implies: "I want toys and clothes off the floor so I can vacuum; I want clothes in the wardrobe hung up on hooks or hangers; I want the bed made with no toys other than stuffed animals on it", and so forth. It will be best to write this down if the child can read or to make pictures together if the child cannot read.

Kurt can be allowed input in the tidying up of his room, too. "I want to be able to keep my cars in the wardrobe, not in the toy basket", or, "I want hooks instead of hangers to put my clothes on because they are easier for me. I do not want you reminding me every day about my room. I'll tidy up on Sundays for the week."

Of course, much of this is negotiable, and again it depends upon the age and stage of your child/family, but this is a broad example of what can be adapted to meet each family's needs. It can also be a means of adapting the environment to meet the child's abilities rather than mandating that the child do something that is beyond his/her capabilities. If Kurt is very unlikely to tidy up his room, perhaps it is best to start just with bed-making. "I would like your bed made and no toys on or under it."

The reward for the clean room, or the bed made, must be agreed upon by both parties, so that parents / carers are not rewarding with something that is actually not gratifying to the child. Similarly, the child cannot be allowed to demand something outrageous as a reward. Just as punishments must only meet the crime, rewards must be kept in proportion, too.

Immediacy is a factor for all ADHD people of any age. A very interesting research experiment (De Posada & Singer, 2005) verified how immediate gratification is a vital part of the ADHD person's life.

The experiment entailed a session with five-year-old children who individually visited an adult. The adult then told the child that she needed to leave the room for a few minutes. She placed a marshmallow on the table and said that the child could eat it while she was gone if the child wanted to, but if the child waited without eating the marshmallow until the experimenter returned, the child could then have two marshmallows.

There were very, very few children with ADHD who managed to wait, while a significantly larger number of non-ADHD children did wait so that they could have two marshmallows. The experiment was a longitudinal one, so that five and ten years later, a similar experiment was conducted with the same subjects. The results were markedly similar.

The point is that even when people with ADHD / ADD know that they can have a bigger or larger or better reward if they wait for it, these individuals still find that they are unable to delay gratification. They say things like, "I know it would have been nicer to have two, but I just couldn't wait," or "I wanted to wait, but I'm so impulsive that I had to have it now."

Motivation

Reinforcement, to some extent, is always an element in our determination of whether or not we choose to do something, but other qualities of the individual, like temperament, disposition, self-confidence, and motivation enter into the equation too. Behaviour can only change when the individual is motivated to make the change, for whatever positive or negative reason that may entail.

Moreover, people like to be consulted about the reward at hand so that they can make a determination about their desire for it. If your employer offers you £10 per hour for your work and you are used to receiving £5 per hour, then it is a good deal; but if you are accustomed to £20, the pay will not be highly motivating. There may be some other reason to accept the job anyway, but the financial reimbursement will not be the motivator. Children who are offered chocolate, or money, or toys, when what they really want is more individual time with a parent, will not find the chocolate/money/toy reinforcement worth their effort.

Although most children like to please adults, many adopted/looked after children have not found this to be a worthwhile form of behaviour, so they are actually no longer motivated to please. In their past experience, they may have tried for a long time to do what mum asked of them or to be very undemanding, but if this behaviour met with disappointment and avoidance or neglect, then there is no desire to repeat that behaviour. Moreover, if a child has been sexually abused, there is virtually no desire (although possibly a lot of fear) to please an adult. Children with these kinds of experiences will become increasingly motivated to behave in a way that pleases themselves, which may entail not doing chores at home, not being polite, not sharing toys, and so forth.

Similarly, ADHD/ADD children usually like to please others, but if the required behaviour is too stressful and/or if there is more gain in not doing something rather than doing it, then they will prefer not to please. Adopted/looked after ADHD/ADD children are so used to getting things wrong or muddled up that they frequently are scared of doing something right because the expectation of their repeating that behaviour is too great. It is easier for them just to keep doing it wrong. These children often seem to be very "defeatist" youngsters, and it is quite a big job to change them around.

Motivation is an important part of how each of us behaves and responds. In adjusting the environment to meet the child's needs, it is important to think about creating an environment in which children feel they can succeed. Many adopted/looked after children and plenty of children with attention problems without hyperactivity have chosen the route of withdrawal. It is often what appears to them to be a safer route. "If I don't do it, I can't fail." "If

I withdraw, I am less likely to be noticed, hurt, humiliated." The experience of these children is that non-involvement is a safer fork in the road. It may be true that they are "lacking in motivation", but, evidently, the environment has not been adequately motivating for them to want to be engaged. ADD children are often quiet dreamers who live in their own worlds. For this reason, they are easily confused with those on the autistic/Asperger's spectrum (a diagnosis which is sometimes as difficult to make as is ADHD/ADD). It is troublesome to watch an infant or toddler go into this shut-down mode. Children who are bored because there is nothing for them to play with, children who have been traumatized, and children who have become disassociated may seem fine for a period of time, and then all of a sudden something happens which triggers old responses in them, and they just "go away". Sometimes they literally fall asleep.

Providing small rewards for taking small risks within the context of the home may be one way of altering the environment to motivate the quiet and withdrawn child. Perhaps you have a neighbour or a relative whom your child likes. Ask that person to come over for a meal and ask your child to help you make a special salad or dessert—or even just a cup of coffee—for the person. In a very low-key fashion, you can then comment,

"Gran, Jenny made this salad for you because I told her how much you like avocados."

Gran should be forewarned not to make a huge deal of this, but to acknowledge Jenny's salad with true appreciation. "Thank you, Jenny. I do like avocados and this is delicious." Maybe Gran could write Jenny a thank you note afterwards. Jenny may choose to throw this away or to treasure it for a long time to come.

It also may turn out that poor old Gran will never come to your house again without being given Jenny's avocado salad, but that's how it goes.

No matter how high the stakes, none of us will be motivated to do something we truly cannot do, and the result is only anxiety. If I am colour-blind, I simply cannot be asked to match up the coloured bricks. The more I am put in this situation, the worse I feel about myself. Offering me £20 to put them in the right baskets is not going to make me any more successful, only more annoyed and disappointed in myself.

The ADHD child in the care system may be able to sit still for five minutes, but not for an hour. This child may be able to remember one task the parent required, but not a whole series of tasks. Children in these categories do very poorly in group situations, while they flourish in one-to-one settings. Making the environment more comfortable for the children can increase their capacity and their desire to concentrate, to learn and to change.

Going out and about

We have all been in restaurants, supermarkets, cinemas, and other public places with screaming children, frantic parents, harsh comments from onlookers, and our own negative thoughts about the child, the parent, the situation. These are not pleasant or easy times for any of those involved.

It probably cannot be repeated too many times: children with attention disorders do not cope with crowds. Sometimes, a crowd is anything more than two people, as in the old adage of two being company and three being a crowd. It is usually a question of over-stimulation. People who have trouble with concentration and focus tend to be very easily over-stimulated. Too many words on a page, noises in the background, people in a place, thoughts to think, lights to look at . . .

Going shopping, to public events, to large parties, to amusement parks and other places that parents would like to think of as fun for their children might actually be creating the fire-breathing dinosaur. There are easier and quieter times one can spend with one's child. For example, you as a parent or carer know that a large department store can be hard to manage because there is too much of everything and the ADHD child will get confused about what to look at, which direction to turn in, or what to buy. It is best not to put the child in the environment that you already anticipate will cause difficulties. As an important aside, adopted/looked after children in a department store may be anxious about getting lost, or they may be tempted to steal, or worried about going in the changing room to try on clothes.

If and when one has a choice, it is highly recommended that ADHD/ADD adopted/looked after children not be taken to settings that can readily over-stimulate them. Of course, there are routine trips to the supermarket that cannot be avoided. Even going to school is a setting that is much too much for many of these children, which is why so many of them do poorly at school. (See Chapter Four.)

If you have other children with you when you go to public places, you will know before you even leave your house that the outing is likely to be problematic. ADHD children are the ones who own every window seat in the car, so just getting to where you are going starts out with difficulties. Zooming up and down grocery store aisles is sheer delight, the excitement being that much greater if a few tins happen to fall off the shelves while you are doing your zooming. When mother puts you in the trolley, it is an excellent time to announce to the entire store that she is unfair and treating you badly, and if you are adopted, this is the ideal moment to scream that she is not your real mother anyway! Being threatened that you will not get your chocolate bar on the way out is your perfect opportunity to tell mum that you don't care, and besides, you don't even like chocolate any more.

It would be very unfair to pretend that there are magical methods of managing this behaviour. On the other hand, there are a few things one can do to try to make it better, and over time, one will see improvement, but, in my experience, there is no magic in this game. What you would do *ideally* can rarely be managed *realistically*, because few people have the time or resource luxury to do the things that would actually make a significant difference. For example, if one parent/carer could take the child in question to the shop alone and pick up one or two items and leave, all in about five minutes, that would be a good first step. In this fantasy scenario, talking to the child beforehand to describe the anticipated event would be useful.

"Sophie, we are going in the car to the supermarket. When we get there, you can choose the kind of bread we buy and I will buy milk. After we pay for the bread and milk, we will get back in the car, and drive home."

Perhaps the child will want to take a toy or a book to have in the car. Let the child choose. Also, letting the child choose the bread—even if you buy another loaf of the kind of bread you want—gives Sophie something to focus on and to do. Maybe she could eat a piece of her chosen bread in the car on the way home.

So, the above is the ideal world that most of us will never experience. In the real world, you are in a hurry, you have a week's worth of grocery shopping to do, and you have two other children with you. If there is a child who is old enough to stay at home with the ADHD child, but who would be helpful in the shop too, I would opt for leaving them both at home. I would also "reward" (pay!) the older child to do this. If, however, all of the children need to go with you, it is actually quite helpful if you have "assigned seats" in the car that are regularly rotated. It can help to have something to play with or read in the car. Giving each child a list of items to look for in the supermarket, or a single item to pick out with you when you get to that aisle, does work. Giving the child, depending upon age, a choice as to riding in the trolley or walking next to you might be a possibility. Give all of the children a small reward when they arrive home if everyone has acted decently, and none of the children a reward if one or more of them have not acted appropriately.

One way of getting other children in the family to work with you instead of scapegoating the ADHD child is to get them used to the fact that rewards are for everyone or no one. When this is the case, they get out of the habit of picking on the ADHD child and/or blaming everything on that child. Rather, they make more of an effort to help, because if they do not tease Sophie and she does not yell and scream and make a fuss, then everyone will get their biscuit, but if she does do those things, then no one will.

At home or out in public, it is a bit of respite for the adult in charge if that person can count on others to help. Rotating this job among other children in the family, and rewarding them for it, is one way of getting some minimal relief. Suppose you are at the cinema and there is a long queue at the ticket counter. Ask Robert to take Steven to the loo and then to look at the video games, where you will meet them—because you already know that there is no way Steven is going to stand in that long queue properly. If Robert manages to do what he was asked to with Steven, surreptitiously give him an extra handful of popcorn and thank him for doing such a good job, or allow both boys to play one video game. This is not bribery; it is rewarding positive behaviour, and it allows you a much more pleasant afternoon.

Thinking about each and every situation in which you will find yourself with a child who does not adapt well is worth the time.

Planning ahead about how you can handle the situation and what will be best for you, for the child, for all of the children or other people involved is time very well spent. Avoiding large crowds and big places and surprises is always going to work better. When possible, giving the child a choice about going or not going, and making clear what the expectations of each choice are will help.

> There is Thursday night dinner at Uncle Bob's. You say to Evan, "If you choose to go to Uncle Bob's with us, you may take some books or toys with you, but you must be prepared to play with them on your own because the rest of us will be talking with Uncle Bob. You must sit with us at the table for at least fifteen minutes before you excuse yourself to play. On the other hand, if you choose to stay home, I will get a baby-sitter and you can play games with her, but no TV. At 8.00 p.m. you need to be in bed."

Then you should also point out what will happen in both of these situations if the child does not do what is expected.

> "If you don't manage your behaviour at Uncle Bob's as we've discussed, then next time, you won't have the choice about going." "If the baby-sitter tells me that you turned the TV on, you won't be able to watch at all this weekend."

Once again, this is giving the child a choice, a choice with consequences, and there are just a couple of very specific behaviours that are being addressed. There is cause and consequence previewed and there must be consistency in the follow-up. The child is given an opportunity to take some control of his own behaviour, and he is reassured that you will be taking control if he should not be able to do what he has agreed to.

None of this is going to work on the first try, and most of it will not even work by the third or fourth try. The adopted/looked after child will not trust you, and the ADHD/ADD child will not remember what you said, which is why it is good to write it down and revisit it afterwards. After lots of trials, however (and lots of errors, it is important to add), some of what you do will begin to have positive results. In time, the adopted/looked after child will come to realize that you are reliable and that you will do what you say you are going to do. If you do the same thing over and over enough times, the ADHD/ADD child's brain begins to recognize a pattern and the repeated behaviours may gel. When trust and neurology work together, change can take place.

There are many aspects of daily living that are difficult for the ADHD/ADD adopted/looked after child and that child's parents and care-takers. There is getting up in the morning, cleaning teeth, getting dressed, eating breakfast, getting everything ready for school, and on and on. All of that is even before 8:00 a.m.! Keeping routines routine, keeping them simple and maintaining extreme patience probably help most. There is certainly something to be said for repetition in the learning process.

A mother of two adopted children told me that she does not mind the erratic behaviour or the forgetfulness or the "jumping about behaviour" nearly as much as she minds the tantrums. "It is the tantrums I can't deal with," she says. Many would agree with her. ADHD adopted/looked after children can flare up so quickly, can be so volatile, can appear so totally irrational in their responses to situations. Their moods and reactions swing back and forth so quickly. Interestingly, they usually recover from their tantrum as quickly and easily as they began it, which is long before the adult in charge has a chance to regain his/her own balance.

Parents, carers, and teachers often report that the child will be absolutely fine two seconds after a half-hour blow-up, and expects the adult to be all sweet and calm then too. The adult, however, is still reeling and disequilibriated, not feeling ready to give hugs or to "make up" quite so quickly. The child usually does not understand why, because he is just fine, thank you: "I'm being nice now."

It is frequently when the child feels that he is being prevented from doing something that he wants to do that aggressive behaviour emerges. The child's intention is strong. When this drive is obstructed, anger kicks in. Ritchie says, "I can't stand it when someone tells me not to do something. It doesn't matter what it is; but I hate being told not to do it. Then I just can't control myself and I go ballistic."

Since these are not children who cope with the detour concept, they tend to see only the goal-post, never any alternative routes of reaching the goal.

Edward (eighteen years old) tells me, "It doesn't matter how you get there. It's just getting there that counts."

I ask Edward what he thinks about the idea of finding happiness in the journey as opposed to just "winning the game".

He answers: "Bullshit! That might be true for others, but not for people like me."

Variations on a theme

Obviously, a big problem for the category of children being discussed is getting them to focus their attention on the proper task at the right time. This is less of a specific behavioural issue than it is one of teaching the child how to focus. I recently spent time with a toddler who is neither adopted nor ADHD, but his inability to pay attention to very much of anything was rather discouraging. This child reflects today's culture of too much television watching, of large day care centres in which there is not enough adult time available to devote to individual children, of too many battery-operated toys that don't require children to figure out how to play creatively or imaginatively with the article. A considerable amount of research, and even the popular press, suggest that the long hours children spend in front of the television or on video games, where they watch extremely fast-paced action and have no verbal or relationship interaction with the entertainment, limits their ability to focus and to formulate well thought out strategies for problem solving.

Some board games help children to learn to strategize and to think about an alternative plan. Draughts and chess are examples of such games. It is also helpful to teach your child mental games that require concentration—like Memory and Kim's Game (see Table 3). In addition, there are also many other commercial and therapeutic games that emphasize the need to plan one's next move in order to have a better chance of reaching one's goal. Moreover, the better games in this genre are set up so that a player's moves affect what other players feel or do. A Year 4 teacher once pointed out to me that the best games to play are those that also have an element of luck in them because it evens the chances for everyone to be able to win and it represents real life. In these games, cognitive ability helps, although it is not always the deciding factor. In my view, that is a concept well worth keeping in mind.

Table 3. Ideas about how to help children attend and focus.

- Use any made-up or commercially produced games requiring memory:
    - For very little children: hide a toy under one of three cups. Ask the child to find it.
    - Memorize poems, definitions of new words, colours of the rainbow.
    - Tell your child three words and ask the child ten minutes later what the words are that you said to remember.
    - Play the card game Memory, Kim's Game, hand-clapping games whose actions go with rhymes or songs.
    - Learn a song—music and words.
- Experiment with various background noise levels to accompany homework or study. Quiet is not always the best. Music can relax.
- Use games and activities that require the child to put together or construct something, such as puzzles, Lego, Duplo, bricks. Practise:
    - colouring inside the lines, stringing beads of different sizes;
    - using nail varnish, almost all art activities, cooking.
- Involve the child in activities that use the whole body and require attention, such as swinging on a swing, playing tag, balancing, climbing, skipping rope, playing jacks, various relay races, most sports, dance, karate.
- Books: *Where's Waldo* and other similar books in which the child has to look for something specific.
    - Find specific words on a page.
    - Listen to a story read by a parent/carer or sibling.
    - Do mazes and word searches (only if the child does not have visual processing difficulties; otherwise these are too frustrating).

The underlying concept of behaviour management, no matter what approach is being followed, is basically a philosophy or approach to child rearing that must be ever-present even though it does not see such immediate results as do specific behaviour modification star charts and games. It is an approach that entails a longer term learning process. In essence, over time, parents want to help their children become independent, so the goal is actually to teach the child to become self-sufficient and to be able to manage his/her own behaviour. At first, it is true, parents and carers need to manage a young child's behaviour, which they do by teaching rules and modelling ways of interacting and setting limits. Gradually, it is hoped that the child will be able to accept a more responsible role in self-conduct. Children with attention difficulties and those whose early life experiences have not taught them the first steps and stages of behaviour regulation will be poorer than others in taking on this responsibility, but that does not mean that they never will do so.

Although cause and consequence generally has little meaning to this group of children, understanding the implications for themselves and others of their actions is eventually what will enable them to become responsible for their own behaviour. Learning this is not an overnight accomplishment and is not taught by tangible reinforcement alone. It is a more subtle process and it has a more individual and unique outcome. Parents and carers do need to discipline their children carefully with both positive and negative reinforcers, but recent research suggests that altering the neurological connections may enable behaviour to derive its own internal rewards rather than relying on external reinforcers. Much of this can be augmented and enhanced by principles used by occupational therapists who are well trained in sensory integration.

For example, the rapid development in brain research has made us aware that the brain affected by early trauma and deprivation recovers most effectively by relearning through experience rather than through "talk therapy". Art, drama, play, and dance therapies have been especially helpful because the actual sensory and physical involvement in these activities is what helps to rewire the brain. Talk therapy requires a certain cognitive and verbal ability, but if a brain is fragile in speech and language, it will not be able to produce enough of the required material to enable a response. Movement therapies are less specifically demanding and more fluid. They encompass a broader range of responses, so painting, drawing, playing, dancing, and acting allow the whole body to be involved in the activity. This is a closer representation of how the young baby acquires new skills and increases brain function in the first place. We do not expect infants to talk, but we do encourage them to move and explore and interact with their environment. Speech follows a bit later on when other neural pathways have become more developed.

Behaviour management strategies at home and in the community that rely on total body involvement and that encourage self-determination—but also provide rewarding experiences and outcomes—are probably the most effective ones to try with adopted/looked after children who have ADHD/ADD. They must all start small, just as one would with a baby, and increase gradually, only as the child shows readiness to move ahead. This can well take a much longer time than anyone would think or hope.

Throughout this process, using some cognitive and psychodynamic techniques may help too. It is the combination of all of these techniques that works best, but getting the balance right is not an easy thing to do.

In summary, the various lists of techniques for management that are suggested throughout this chapter must be read within the context that the chapter has been written. That is to say, they are not presumed to be magic and they are not assumed to work for everyone. They are kick-off points to generate some ideas of where one might start and what some people have found to be helpful. A really useful and relevant technique is talking with friends, colleagues, and professionals about what they have tried, discarded, found helpful, benefited from. Many of the suggestions do come from parents and children, who are sometimes better than professionals at devising strategies that really do work. Again, the combination of research based knowledge and practical experience will provide the most effective means of dealing with these challenges.

CHAPTER FOUR

The ADHD/ADD adopted/ looked after child at school

Daniel has already been to four different schools in his young life. He has not been to school regularly though, and is not sure just what he is supposed to do in a classroom because all his schools and teachers have been so different. Daniel can remember his last school because he had a nice teacher who didn't mind when he looked out of the window a lot. She also let him clean the blackboards at lunch-time when he didn't want to stay out on the playground. In his first school, Daniel knew one other girl because she was in foster care with him. They were allowed to sit next to each other in class when Daniel wasn't sitting by himself for being in trouble for his behaviour or for talking when he wasn't supposed to. He doesn't remember the next school because he wasn't allowed to go there for very long. He says, "I talked too much and threw too many pencils at that school."

Christie's school experiences have been equally inconsistent, although for the most part she has worked out how to be the "kid in the corner" that nobody pays attention to. Christie doesn't actually pay much attention either because she doesn't understand a lot of what is being taught, and she finds it hard to keep her mind on what the teacher is talking about. She likes numbers, though, as they make more sense to her, so she does well in maths and sometimes even raises her hand to volunteer an answer during maths class. Christie finds it hard to make friends at school and rarely has anyone to be with at playtime. She says, "I suppose I don't know what to say to anyone."

Attention deficits are among the most common sources of maladaptive behaviour during the school years. Affected children exhibit a wide range of characteristics that directly or indirectly reflect difficulties controlling thought processes and behaviours. Few children have insight into the condition of attention deficit, but they do know that they are always getting into trouble and that their attention difficulties interfere with their schoolwork. They recognize that it is hard for them to make and keep friends, although they almost always see this as the other person's fault. As ADHD/ADD adopted/looked after children fall further behind academically and socially in school, they begin to lose interest, completing fewer and fewer assignments and paying even less attention. Problems with oppositional behaviour arise as the child and teacher fall into patterns of negativity.

In Chapter One, it was pointed out that the behaviour of ADHD children is predictably unpredictable. Even so, it can be anticipated that, on most days, these are not going to be easy children to have in one's classroom. The same may or may not be the case for adopted and looked after children, who sometimes do better at school than anywhere else in their lives. On the other hand, ADHD/ADD adopted/looked after children more than likely have caused one or two disruptions in previous schools or classrooms, and it is highly possible that their school careers have not been entirely productive experiences for them or for their teachers.

The statistics relating to looked after children and their educational attainment are categorically dismal. In this group of youngsters there are more learning difficulties, more bullying and being bullied, more school drop-outs, more teenage pregnancies, and higher rates of later incarceration than among any other minority group (The Who Cares? Trust, 2003). Educational vulnerability puts a great burden on the child, but it also becomes a difficult task for the teachers responsible for the child.

Although the government has recently been more attentive to improving the education of looked after children, only small steps have been taken. The White Paper, *Care Matters* (DfES, 2007), does put into place the expectation that children in care will be given the highest priority in school admission arrangements, and that care planning decisions will not disrupt a child's education, especially in Years 10 and 11. There are proposals to issue strengthened guidance to carers and those with parental responsibility for children with special educational needs; clauses that provide for extra money for children in care who are at risk for not attaining the expected targets; and provisions for reducing school absence and exclusion. Nevertheless, these aspirations have yet to be tried and tested, and the history up until the White Paper uniformly confirms that looked after children do not do well in school (Comfort, 2007; Geddes, 2006; Jackson, 2001, 2007; Jackson & McParlin, 1998).

Once children are adopted, they are more likely to have a smoother course of education, as it is less probable that they will change schools so frequently. Furthermore, they may have better access to diagnostic educational assessments, and they will usually have more consistent input from their adoptive parents than they would have had while moving from foster home to foster home and from school to school. Subsequent to adoption, and depending upon the age at which they are adopted and their previous school experiences, their educational careers may have a better chance of taking off in a positive direction.

The degree to which the child's attention disorders have been assessed and diagnosed will influence how well the child manages at school too. Adopted/looked after children sometimes have so many overwhelming emotional difficulties that it is not always possible to tease out just what is a clinical attention deficit and what appears to be an attention disorder. This differentiation, however, is actually less important than one might assume, because both adopted and looked after children and ADHD/ADD children need particular educational and behavioural management approaches that often can be combined and worked on simultaneously, although there are exceptions to this rule. It is also important to assess whether there are attachment difficulties and/or other specific learning disorders that are influencing the child's educational, social–emotional and behavioural functioning that make the child appear to be ADHD/ADD when he or she is not.

If the child suffers any one of a number of processing disorders or speech/language dysfunctions, for example, the teacher needs to be aware of that because these must be treated as entities unto themselves. Usually, addressing and correcting, or even modifying, a specific learning disorder in a non-ADHD/ADD student will enable the child to focus and attend to classroom learning much more effectively.

Since most children spend about six hours a day at school, it puts teachers in a powerful position to have an important effect on a child's life (both positively and negatively, it must be pointed out). The child with a troubled background, with attention difficulties, and possibly with other learning disorders as well, is likely to be a child with a defeatist attitude about school and is one who can ignite a lot of fire in a short period of time. However, the gratification for a teacher who turns this child around will be immense, and the child will never forget such an important person.

On the other hand, some children in the care system will have had a positive school experience, and these children may be able to put some of their concerns aside during the school day while they make every effort possible to focus on the teacher and on learning. Many of these children may not be children with a clinical attention deficit, but those whose emotional backgrounds make them highly distractible in the classroom. If school has been the "safe" place for them, they will do better here than they do at home or in the community.

Almost every adult who was abused in childhood and who has come through it to live a productive life will say that there was one person who believed in them and pulled them through. Not very surprisingly, most of the time this person was a teacher. Periodically, looked after children who had horrendous early years and massive disruption in their lives will talk about a teacher who stood by them and encouraged them to want to learn so they could get ahead in life.

> Lydia is twenty-seven years old. She left home at eleven and dropped out of school at thirteen, getting into drugs and street life while moving in and out of numerous foster homes. Through amazing determination and a stroke of luck, she pulled herself through and now manages a small electrical company. When asked about her early life, she says, "I had such low expectations of myself; I was lonely and angry. I had trouble focusing in school and probably had all of those things they talk about now . . . ADHD or whatever. You know, I didn't fit in or anything. My home was so chaotic. Other kids went home and did

homework and had some organization in their lives, but I didn't have that. My dad was an alcoholic and there was so much verbal abuse all of the time."

When asked about her second chance in life and how it came about, she replies immediately:

"Reading saved me! I was so naughty in the classroom that the teacher sent me to the library for punishment all of the time. The library teacher was cool. She gave me lots and lots of books to read and I behaved beautifully with her. She always asked me about the books and we talked together. If it weren't for that library teacher, I'm sure I'd still be on the streets."

For some adopted and looked after children, the school environment does feel safer and easier than the child's home. This is not a reflection on the foster or adoptive family, but on the past experience of the child for whom family life has not been as rewarding as school life. If a child from a dysfunctional family, or a child who has been moved from home to home, has had the unusually good fortune to stay in the same school, and it was one he liked and in which he was doing well, he may encounter academic and social success that defies his difficult background. Maybe this child made a friend at school—his only friend ever. Maybe the child was chosen for the cricket team and earned a school-wide reputation as an outstanding athlete. Maybe a lot of things, or maybe not. Whatever the book of maybes, it will have significantly influenced how a child feels about school, about learning, about how he will or can behave in school. Peter is an example of how things can work out well.

Peter is ten years old. A large boy for his age, he has been able to hold his own at school in spite of having difficulties with attention and with reading. Peter is an outstanding athlete and he excels in drama—strengths that have stood him in good stead among his peers, who don't really mind that he doesn't read very well, and who are amused by his ADHD because he is funny and makes the class laugh. Peter has moved families four times, but only made one school change. Although he is not an easy child to manage in the classroom, his teachers tend to like him, too, because he is creative and he means well. He talks out of turn a lot and frequently gets out of his seat, but he is never rude or mean.

For most ADHD/ADD adopted/looked after children though, just being among so many others and trying to comply with school and social rules can be too much to handle. Real or perceived pressures and interruptions that come into play throughout the school day can be terribly distracting for these children. It has been said that the way schools are constructed and boys are made is not a good fit. Perhaps the same pertains to children who have attention difficulties, and for children who have issues other than school work on their minds.

What ADHD/ADD adopted/looked after children may have trouble doing

- Staying in their seats, or even in the designated part of the classroom.
- Choosing the right piece of information on which to concentrate.
- Staying focused on the right information for the right amount of time.
- Filtering out distractions.
- Coping with details.
- Following a series of instructions or a sequence of directions.
- Planning and monitoring their work and behaviour.
- Not talking or behaving impulsively.

How hard it can be to teach!

Teachers are in a difficult position because each teacher has a room full of very different personalities and abilities and needs. Often, teachers say that they do not have time to teach thirty students in thirty different ways, and certainly no one is going to argue with the fact that teachers do require monumental patience and endurance day after day. Interestingly, though, adjusting to the needs of the students is often easier than dealing all day long with a chaotic or ill-behaved group of children. Fortunately, many of the approaches to learning and behaviour management that work well for ADHD/ADD adopted/looked after children work well for everyone in the classroom, and nothing that works well for them can be harmful to any other child. On the other hand, these youngsters can distract not only themselves, but other students as well, and their energy levels do demand a certain mental and physical fitness on the part of the teacher.

Even so, there are many small techniques and methods all teachers can employ in virtually any classroom that will reduce the amount of negativity and non-compliance which children with any learning or living disorder are likely to manifest at school.

One very small example of this is the use of carbon paper to help children who have trouble copying from the board or writing down assignments. If Joey has visual or fine motor difficulties (or ADHD/ADD) and never seems to finish writing what is on the board, the teacher can put a piece of carbon paper under the paper of a child who has no trouble writing, and bingo, both children have the assignment written down properly and the teacher did not have to do any extra work at all.

By definition, children with attention difficulties have a disorder that can interfere with educational functioning. After all, it is hard to learn when paying attention is not what you do very well. Paradoxically, though, this is a disorder with somewhat of a misnomer because people with ADHD actually *do* pay attention. What they do is to pay too much attention to everything without knowing what to filter out (Levine, 1987). Their executive functioning in the brain works poorly, meaning that they absorb everything going on around them rather than editing out some of what is irrelevant. Usually, they take things in without knowing what is the important information on which to focus, and this can result in their responding to the wrong subject matter. For example, they see all of the small chalk marks on the board that did not quite get erased; they know the exact route of the ladybird who flew in the open window and is marching across the desk of the girl in the front row; they hear the bell outside that marks the end of playtime for the preschoolers; but they have no clue about what the teacher just told the class to do for homework that night. If asked, "Weren't you listening to me?", this child will say "Yes", and will truthfully have done so. The problem is that the child was listening to about six other things going on in the classroom as well. If the teacher had asked the child if the overhead lights were buzzing, the child would have known the correct answer: "Yes, they were."

How ADHD/ADD adopted/looked after children might feel in school

- Worried that they will not be able to follow the instructions.
- Scared about not being able to get all of their work finished.
- Embarrassed that their work does not look as nice or is "not as good as" most other student's work.
- Concerned that they cannot write down the ideas in their heads.
- Frustrated that they are not able to control their behaviours and moods.
- Afraid that teachers and students will be annoyed with them and will make them annoyed.
- Anxious about losing track, day-dreaming, tuning out, and needing to move around.

When we send ADHD/ADD adopted/looked after children to school, we ask of them something we would never ask of ourselves. Which of us would voluntarily go to a job each day that drew on all of our weaknesses, and offered us very little that we either liked to do or were good at doing? Moreover, at this job, the odds were stacked in favour of our having a boss who felt that if we tried harder, we could do better, and so he either ignored us or was annoyed with us most of the day.

Unintentionally, this is the position we put many ADHD/ADD adopted/looked after children in much of the time. Children are obliged to go to school and to attend to specific subjects at certain times. The ten-year-old is not allowed to say that the spelling test is not on his personal agenda for the day, thank you, and that he will choose to go to the playground instead. As adults, however, people usually choose a job or vocation that better suits their needs.

> I sat in a coffee shop the other day, trying to do some work, but was continuously distracted by listening to and watching a waitress there. "What a perfect job this is for her," I thought to myself because she was clearly a young lady who needed to do some moving about and some chatting. I am sure that this woman would never have "made it" it in an office job where she was made to sit at a desk all day. However, she was a very popular waitress who knew most of the people who came in, delighted in being friendly with them, and then was equally happy

to move about to the next tasks of clearing tables and serving coffees. I felt pleased for her and reminded myself: "There *is* life after school!"

Adults are not required to sit in a classroom all day attending to tasks that draw out all of their weaknesses. Rather, they are given the freedom to choose their own direction and to use their unique style to their distinct advantage. Adults are able to choose jobs and lifestyles that are more likely to meet their individual needs. When they do not do this, they find they either lose the job or that their performance is quite inadequate. Often they become depressed. This can be true for children at school too, and it is especially possible for those children who have any form of a learning disorder or emotional and behavioural difficulties. Not always, but frequently, ADHD / ADD adopted / looked after children fall into this category. It certainly suggests that accommodating the educational programme and environment to the child's specific needs will be reflected in a higher functioning student.

As with everything, children and their experiences and their ways of handling these experiences differ dramatically, but, in general, there are traits and characteristics that tend to hold true. Knowing about the many similarities of ADHD / ADD children and about adopted / looked after children can be beneficial for a teacher because, if nothing else, it can provide a point of entry in dealing with the behaviour. Sometimes it does not work to start at this point, but needing to begin somewhere, it is probably more efficacious to do so with a knowledge base.

Information processing

The process of dealing with information is very much like making something in a blender. It is first necessary to put the ingredients into the blender. Then they have to be mixed up or "blended" in some form or other. Finally, they need to be poured out of the blender. This is essentially what our brains do with information, too. Children with various learning disorders can have a glitch in any part of the blender process, so maybe they do not take the information in correctly (often the case with those having auditory or visual processing difficulties), or maybe they take the information in correctly, but then they have trouble dealing with the material once it has been ingested. This could be seen in children who have memory deficits or children who have attention disorders that inhibit their sorting out and dealing with the important parts of what they have taken in. At length, something must be done with the information in terms of output. In school, this often means writing down one's thoughts and knowledge, telling it to someone, or showing what one has learned by producing a product: a science experiment or a map or a history chart, and so forth.

More often than not, ADHD/ADD adopted/looked after children actually do take in the information, but then they have trouble dealing with it, or, more frequently, they are too impatient or shy or distracted to be able to "show and tell". This aspect of the process is referred to as "Developmental Output Failure". If the child has not taken in the information properly and/or has not dealt with it in a meaningful manner, the output may be inappropriate or incorrect. However, it may be that the child actually has processed the information, but has trouble with the output factor, and therefore responds inappropriately, or does not respond at all. We have all had the experience of not being able to come up with someone's name: we know our friend's name perfectly well, but when starting to introduce the friend to someone new, we all of a sudden completely "forget" the name, which leaves us in a kind of frozen state, not knowing what to say or do next.

The ADHD/ADD adopted/looked after child might often find him/herself at this awkward junction, particularly since attention deficits affect performance, not intelligence. Children who have been abused may shut down upon receiving input if that input seems frightening or worrying to them. It does not actually even have to be the information itself that concerns them. It may be the look on the teacher's face, or the sound of the voice of the supply teacher, or that the information reminds the child of something else. These children may shut down for their own sense of survival; although sometimes it is an almost autonomic response and it occurs before they are conscious of having shut down.

Don't fence me in

ADHD/ADD adopted/looked after children do not like to be confined and restricted. Teachers who have such children in their classrooms do well to allow them a certain amount of choice and flexibility. Even the knowledge that there is some opportunity to choose will often mollify the seemingly obstreperous student. It is being told: "Sit in your chair", "Read this book", "You can't go out to play", etc., which make ADHD / ADD adopted / looked after children scared. Their intense need for "flight" when they feel backed up against the wall can escalate any minor difficulty into one of magnified outrage. Just knowing that they have a way out can calm the situation before it spirals out of control.

> Mr Tom was a brilliant teacher who kept his class of nine-year-olds inspired and invested in learning almost all of the time. He told marvellous stories, and did wonderful science experiments, and made maths magical. What Mr Tom had trouble with, however, was tolerating children who could not comply and could not participate in what he was teaching. His temper was short with such children, and several became quite afraid of him. His student, Oliver, a child who had recently been taken into care and was seen to be quite a distractible lad, told me that he did fine in maths and science and history, but it was too hard for him to listen to Mr Tom's stories because they always seemed to remind him of things he was trying not to think about any more. When Mr Tom asked them to do writing after these stories, Oliver just couldn't do it. Then Mr Tom became very angry with Oliver and that made things get a lot worse. Oliver had several times thrown a chair or threatened others with scissors during these episodes.
>
> When Mr Tom learned about Oliver's situation and his worries over these stories, he gave Oliver the choice of staying in the classroom during story time or of going to the next class where they were having maths lessons. Oliver usually left. His anxiety and the tension in the classroom were enormously diffused—all because Oliver now had a choice and could take control over the situation.

Adopted and looked after children may have extreme and unusual needs when they feel that their "space" is being invaded or when they sense that they are losing control of an uncomfortable situation. Those who have been left alone in cots or strapped into infant seats for long periods of time might have visceral memories of being "stuck" or "trapped". Those who have been mistreated and then left, literally, out in the cold, may sense it is a time to run away or to hide. Children usually will not have the words to articulate any of these sensations because what happened to them was preverbal, but their bodies respond instantly when they feel that they are going to be restricted in some way or another or when they feel that their freedom of choice is being curtailed. Instantaneously, without having a chance to think of anything rational or to think about anyone else, children who have had this past experience lash out in whatever way they feel they need to in order not to be confined (Golding, Dent, Nissim, & Stott, 2006; Heineman, 1998).

Throughout this book, it has been necessary at times to describe the ADHD/ADD child separately from the adopted/looked after child. Despite the fact that there are many overlapping issues, and independent of the scope of the book, which is to look at the adopted/looked after child who has an attention disorder, it is sometimes important to think about their various issues separately. Once in a while, there are behaviour management approaches that would be useful for a child with ADHD, but that would be contraindicated for a child who is or has been in care. So, for example, normally we would think to give a child who has been acting disruptively and inappropriately a period of time out. This is indeed a very feasible response to an ADHD child who needs to be isolated in order to regain control. Adopted/looked after children, however, are often terribly afraid of being isolated because being left alone has so many frightening and miserable associations for them.

Like parents and carers, therefore, teachers are in a bind as to how to make the most beneficial decision about what will be right and effective for the out-of-control student. These situations always come up when there is not a lot of thinking time available and some sort of decision will have to be made quickly. Although a child may need to be removed in order to keep him and others safe, it is best if the adopted/looked after child can be taken out of the situation with a classroom aide, or even with another student he generally considers to be a friend. If the child is sent to the Head Teacher's office, someone should stay close by the child at all times. This accompanying person does not have to talk, or to be a specialist of any kind, but the person should be someone whom the ADHD/ADD adopted/looked after child sees as a friend. It must be remembered that the anger and fear inside this youngster can be so unbearable that reason and thought have absolutely no chance to surface. It is not helpful to try to talk to the child at this time and it is not helpful to try to get him/her to be rational. What the child needs is to feel safe and in control of him/herself. Helping the child to a place of calmness is the most effective method of dealing with this kind of behaviour. Talk, and a review of the situation, can come later—sometimes much later. The child needs to be in a good space in order to be able to look at and to try to understand the outrageous behaviour exhibited earlier on.

Adopted/looked after students with ADHD/ADD generally require a balance of structure and flexibility in the classroom. A dichotomy for both these students and their teachers is that they do need structure and routine, but they also need to be given a fair amount of independence and choice. As has been seen above, it is never worth battling with these children because it is a no-win situation. They may be impulsive, they may be inconsistent, and they may be irrational, but if pushed too hard to do what they do not want to do, ADHD/ADD adopted/looked after children will win all ten rounds in the boxing arena. Subsequently, they and the adult will feel exhausted and deflated, and absolutely nothing will have been gained. Adopted/looked after children with ADHD/ADD do not have flexible characters, and they become even more rigid when pushed, because they are desperately striving to be in control of the situation. Their need to gain control overrides any form of reasoning at the time, although later they may well see things more objectively.

Since none of us can ever really control anyone else, the best we can do in these difficult situations is to try to control ourselves. When a teacher finds herself in a battle with a child, I think it shows reasonableness and good modelling for the teacher to say something like:

> "Dixon, I don't think we are getting anywhere with this discussion. I am going to just leave it now while you and I both take a break. Later, perhaps you will be able to pick up the pencil you have thrown on the floor, or perhaps you won't, but I think we had better drop things now until we both cool down."

This enables both parties to bow out gracefully with no one losing face. Although Dixon may not ever pick up the pencil he threw, because he would see that as giving in, he may be less likely to throw it another time. At the very least, he may be less likely to throw anything else at that moment, or he may throw several more things just to test the teacher.

Bennett is the middle of three boys, all of whom are extremely clever students. Their dad is doing time in prison for drug-related issues and their mother has recently become quite ill physically. Bennett's father has a long history of school exclusions, and ultimately left school and home at fifteen years of age. It is likely that Bennett's dad had specific learning disorders and / or ADHD but was never assessed or diagnosed properly. As is often the case, drugs became an alternative to school and work when he went out on the street. Bennett's parents met during a brief period of dad's sobriety when he was in treatment and she was a summer helper at the facility. Throughout her first pregnancy, their marriage stayed stable, but when she became pregnant with Bennett, things began to fall apart again.

At eight years of age, Bennett has been shown to have an IQ of 147, but he is under-performing at school, and is constantly in trouble. Recently, due to his mother's poor health, he and his younger brother were taken into care, but they are not in the same foster family. It is, of course, rhetorical to say that Bennett is having a horrible time at school now, and his teacher is absolutely beside himself.

Sadly, this is not a terribly unusual scenario. Here is an eight-year-old child who was just barely coping with a very untenable situation at home when things went from pretty awful to really unbearable. Teachers are plunked down with children who are in these scary, worrying, desperate situations, but the teacher has little time to spend individually with such a child, and often does not even know the story behind the child's behaviour.

In Bennett's case, his teacher did know, but he was given no support and no additional training or help as to how he might handle Bennett's emotions and behaviours. At the suggestion of another teacher, Mr Bay decided to ask Bennett to join him for lunch several days a week, and the two of them ate together in the classroom. This gave Bennett some individual attention and it kept him off the playground, which is always the hardest place for children who have trouble controlling their behaviour or understanding the unwritten social rules of what is described as "the killing ground" in the poem, "Back in the Playground Blues" (Mitchell, 1984).

You cannot do it all

Teachers are taught to teach, and it is unfair to expect them to be counsellors as well. Nevertheless, many teachers are faced with very disturbed children, either because of their home and family situations, or because of a variety of learning disorders, one of which may be ADHD / ADD. Both adopted / looked after children and children with ADHD / ADD bring hugely complicated histories with them to school (Cairns, 2002; Fahlberg, 1995; Geddes, 2006). Schools that support and help teachers who have especially involved children in their classrooms are more likely to have teachers, students, and classrooms that function more efficiently than schools who do not have either the personnel or the inclination to provide this kind of input.

On the other hand, teachers and Heads often say that they do not believe in treating children differently: "This is Year 5 and I expect such and such of all of the children in this classroom." Does that teacher also expect the deaf child to hear and the visually impaired child to read what is written on the blackboard? Probably not, so why might the teacher anticipate that the child with learning or living disorders can match the output of students without these difficulties? A fair education is one in which children are treated differently rather than the same. Within this environment of difference, it is also fair to create an atmosphere of respect in which all students and teachers are expected to treat others with tolerance and kindness, but it is unfair to expect each child to think and behave equally.

We so readily make adaptations when there is a physical disability involved, but we often forget to do so when there is "a hidden handicap". Children with an attention deficit do not look any different from other children, any more than adopted / looked after children do, so it can be hard for others to recognize that they might need to be treated differently in some situations. While some adopted or looked after children do show their scars of abuse, most carry them on the inside where they are not easily observed. In fact, it is often only their behaviour that signals something wrong is going on inside them. Children with learning and emotional dysfunctions require special attention just as much as those with physical disabilities do. Treating each student according to his / her needs can diffuse a difficult situation for any individual child and certainly will help to protect the entire class from a frightening or annoying incident.

Realistically, no teacher is ever going to absolutely love all of the children in the classroom year after year. There is always a child or two with whom any of us just cannot cope. As an individual therapist, one has the choice to refer the child elsewhere, but this does not happen much in schools. Every once in a while a teacher can ask to transfer a student out of her classroom, but that is a very rare occasion. It is important for Heads and other school personnel to be receptive to a teacher who is struggling with a student, just as much as it is reasonable to accept that a particular child may be having exceptional difficulties with a given teacher. In either case, both the student and the teacher need to know that there is someone else in the school setting who can be there to help and support them. Children with special needs are sometimes quite astute about sussing out the person who will be receptive to them. This might be a dinner lady, the school nurse, the caretaker, or the teacher the child had last year and with whom he did well. Teachers might look for an empathic ear and for some professional input from an educational specialist.

Issues that may be unique to the adopted/looked after child

When teachers become more aware of what any given child is struggling with, and when they are more attuned to the impairments of a child, they are almost always much more sensitive to and understanding of that child. Very often, I have heard teachers say, "Oh! So that is why she always does such and such . . ." Simply knowing, for instance, that an adopted or looked after child finds the Tuesday afternoon "Contact" with the birth parent enormously stressful will enable the teacher to respond differently than if she thinks the child is just wilfully being obstinate and unco-operative. (Contact is a visit the adopted or looked after child has with a birth relative. The frequency of these visits, and who attends, is usually determined by the court or the social worker.)

If a teacher knows that a Contact visit is coming up or has just occurred, he may decide not to call on this particular child to answer questions that day, recognizing that the child will already be in an uncomfortable state in anticipation of the visit or is having repercussions from the get-together that took place earlier.

Furthermore, this sensitive teacher might decide to have a little chat with the child so the child knows the teacher understands that Contact afternoons are hard times. The teacher can ask the child if she needs some time to herself before or after visits, or if the child would like to have a time set up to talk with the teacher or the school counsellor before or after Contact. Maybe, simply hearing the teacher say he cares will be enough for the child to feel a bit better.

The whole issue of Contact has enormous relevance to the story of any adopted or looked after child, and is another area in which adopted/looked after children with ADHD/ADD differ from ADHD/ADD children who are not or have not been in care (Borkowski, 2007; McCaskill, 2002). In general, Contact in and of itself can make any adopted/looked after child appear to be a student with an attention disorder because the emotions Contact elicits usually have high intensity ramifications. Contact is complex and often contentious, but beyond the scope of this book. In a nutshell, teachers need to know that the days before, of, or after Contact can be extremely difficult ones for an adopted/looked after child, even when the Contact is "good". These children are likely to show exaggerated responses and emotions around the time of Contact, and having ADHD/ADD only makes this harder for them and worse for those around them.

Like Contact, the decision of "To Tell or Not to Tell" is a tricky issue. All adopted or looked after children deal with a situation that children not in care never even think about, and that is the issue of whether they want to tell teachers or friends that they are adopted or looked after. Usually the latter are known to the school because every school is supposed to have a "designated teacher" who is responsible for looked after children, but these are the youngsters who least want anyone to know about their situation. Adopted children sometimes are proud to be adopted and are happy to share that information; at other times they do not want anyone to know anything about it.

Most children do not want to be singled out as being different, but being adopted or looked after already makes a child different from the majority, even though it is becoming more common than it once was. Despite the broad mixtures of families in today's world, looked after children in particular, and adopted children to some extent, still feel stigmatized by society. If things are generally going well for these children at school, they may see "telling" others as a way of jeopardizing their relationships with them, whether it be teachers or friends.

There are also issues for children looked after or adopted of what the child has left behind and about whom that child might be worried. Adopted and looked after children carry a huge history of experiences that the vast majority of their peers will never know about in their own lives or even be able to consider that some other child is dealing with on a day to day basis. For instance, most young children do not experience severe physical abuse or sexual abuse, so these are concepts that do not come into their knowledge base until they are quite a bit older. The fact that their five-, six-, or seven-year-old peers might have this kind of story to tell never even occurs to them.

> Betsy is a nine-year-old who was adopted at six years of age. She talks to me about her worry that others will find out she is adopted. "My brother told his best friend that he was adopted and some other boy overheard him and then told everyone else around what he had heard. I'm afraid of that. I only want certain people to know, but I don't know if I can trust them not to say anything."
>
> Karen agrees. She is an eleven-year-old in foster care. "Yeah, that happened to me. I told my best friend and she blabbed it to the whole school. Now she's not my friend any more, but still everyone knows."

The concern for these children and the many others in their situation is that they will get teased or bullied, and that others will find out things about them. If these children are ADHD, they are likely to blurt out information about themselves, and then regret having done so. Maybe it feels acceptable to have ADHD, but it is not acceptable to be in care or to be adopted. The horrible fear of hearing "Your mother didn't want you," is enough to keep many of these children from paying attention to almost anything that the teacher is teaching.

These children worry about their birth families, about social workers and police, about whether or not their new family will keep them or move them, about having enough food, about where and how their siblings are, about safety, about being "found out", about keeping up. The litany goes on and on. That is a lot of worry for both them and their teachers to contend with, and it is certainly a heavy enough burden to make any child distractible.

> Bradley is a twelve-year-old boy whom I have known since he was three years old. He has been in and out of more foster homes than any child I've ever met, but has lived in a long-term placement for the past three years. With great credit to an amazing foster parent, this placement is destined to hold.
>
> Bradley has a lot of relatives in town. He also knows a large number of children around the city from having been in foster care with them, and because of changing schools so frequently.
>
> On several occasions, I have taken Bradley out to an event or an activity in the city, and he inevitably runs into at least three or four youngsters or adults whom he knows. When I've asked him if he likes seeing so many people who are contacts from the past, he always beams and says that he does.
>
> On the other hand, Bradley and I have talked quite a bit about school, which is a difficult place for him, and about friends there, because at his current school there is a half-brother of his in his class and two children whom he knew from previous foster placements. "We keep it quiet," Bradley tells me. "No one is going to rat on you because we are all the same. There's nothing in it for anyone to say anything about you since it is saying the same thing about them. I know; they know; finished."
>
> "Finished" is about the length of conversation we have on this topic, too. It is definitely not a subject that Bradley wants to pursue.

Parents and carers, especially long-term carers, also wonder if they should tell or not tell. Some parents will tell teachers that their child is adopted and some will give a bit of history that is deemed important for the teacher to know, but parents worry about the same things that their children do, namely: can the parent trust the teacher to maintain confidentiality and trust. Without knowing a teacher's own views about adoption and fostering, how much risk does the parent want to take? In fairness, most teachers do handle this information appropriately and judiciously, but there certainly have been instances when that is not the case.

On the positive side, if a parent or carer has shared information with the teacher about either adoption and fostering or an attention deficit, the teacher is then in a good position to ask the parent or carer for help. Parents and carers often know a lot about "what works" with their child, and anything that is effective at home and can be replicated at school is money in the bank. It is also extremely helpful if teachers can learn from parents/carers about specific things that may upset the child.

One example of this is that many adopted/looked after children are very afraid of a banging door. This often signifies upcoming adult fighting and/or neglect of the child. These children, and especially those who also have ADHD, will hear that door slamming much more readily than will anyone else in the classroom. It does not have to be their classroom door; it can well be a door far down the corridor! Just the sound of the slamming door can quickly put the child in a state of panic or withdrawal or aggression that was not aroused half a minute before the door banged. The teacher might feel that the child became aggressive (or passive) "for no reason", and the teacher will not understand why the child all of a sudden lashed out (or withdrew). Interestingly, the child may not know at a very conscious level either. How much easier it would be if this child could simply say, "I am afraid of slamming doors because when my dad slammed the door at home it always meant a fight and then we kids didn't get fed for a long time." This is not the way it works though. Usually, the child does not quite know what happened, but may be able to say that she got scared or a sick feeling came over her. More often, hurt or angry children do not connect any of these feelings and cannot say anything at all about why their behaviour changed, but they do feel something foreboding or reminiscently uncomfortable inside of them.

Although teachers do well to ask parents/carers about their children, and although it may sometimes be useful to ask the child about how he is feeling, teachers should not expect that young children are going to put two and two together at an emotional level. Most children do not do this very well anyway, but those who have been traumatized hide things away in very deep cupboards, and children do not like to go searching in deep, dark cupboards. Unfortunately, the ghosts emerge from time to time despite the child's desires (some of them emerge pretty frequently), and then both the child and the teacher (and the rest of the classroom) may be looking at very scary feelings that no one wants to touch. In order to hide feelings, and often because both ADHD / ADD and adopted / looked after children can be quite creative, the child may tell stories that actually have no bearing on reality at all, or that may be the child's perceived view of the reality. Sometimes, however, they are just amazingly wonderful fantasies that the child wants to tell and wants someone else to believe. Moral of the story: teachers, do not discount what a child is telling you, but do not believe everything you hear either.

Patterns of behaviour

When referring to ADHD / ADD adopted / looked after children, there is going to be quite a large continuum on which any given student may reside behaviourally and emotionally. Moreover, it is very likely that this child will see-saw all over the spectrum, depending upon the day and what is going on in the rest of the child's life at the moment. While this is true of all children, youngsters in the specified category we are discussing tend to be quite a bit more extreme than other children. They do not necessarily do anything that is particularly different from other children (although they might). Usually they just do what other children do, but they do it to the extreme.

Rather than becoming annoyed with a child who seems to have acted out irrationally, it is quite a bit more interesting for a teacher to look at seemingly irrational or aberrant behaviour in an objective manner and wonder about what could have instigated the reaction in the child that the teacher observed. It helps to diffuse the anger and frustration for the teacher when this approach is taken, because it becomes more of a problem-solving effort instead of a disciplinary issue. "I wonder what just happened for James that I didn't notice, but that caused him to become so upset all of a sudden", is a calmer and more introspective method of dealing with the problem. It may be possible to ask James, or it may just be a key to the teacher that James needs a safety net around him for a few minutes. This would be a good time to give James a break and then to refocus him on something that he usually does well. Teachers who become invested in the nuances and particularities of their children can be enormously helpful to the child and to the parents/carers. Seeing behaviour as a symptom that is similar to a learning disability or to a physical impairment can make the teacher become more intrigued with ideas for developing creative strategies to help the child in question.

Not all of the children's behaviours are going to be inexplicable, though. Some of them are just annoying, or perfectly rational but hard to manage. Table 4 is a condensed list of patterns of behaviours that teachers and schools might expect to experience in ADHD/ADD adopted/looked after children. Most of the children will not do all of these things all of the time, but any of these problematic behaviours could be manifested throughout any given day. The child's lack of appreciation of cause and consequence as well as the child's impulsivity can contribute to the school day being a challenge for the student as well as for the teacher.

Some strategies that often work, and why they do

In this and previous chapters it has been pointed out that ADHD/ADD adopted/looked after children have a high need for structure and for boundaries. It has also been said many times that consistency and predictability contribute to their home and school success. There is a considerable amount of literature detailing classroom set-up and basic teacher techniques for the management of children with attention difficulties. (See Appendix III.) Among these suggestions, one usually finds the following list of things for the teacher to think about in accommodating the ADHD/ADD child:

- where the child sits;
- breaking the work into small "chunks";
- how much is too much stimulation on the display boards;
- what the personalities and temperaments are of the other children at the work table;
- how often breaks are built in;
- preparing the child for transitions and changes (something this group of children is exceptionally poor at managing).

Table 4. What schools might expect ADHD/ADD adopted/looked after children to find difficult.

Knowing and/or being able to follow the rules of the classroom and the school.
Staying in their seat/
Talking at the allotted time only/
Waiting their turn.
Not needing to be first in the queue every time.
Not speaking out of turn or before being called upon.
Being a good listener.
Being in the right place at the right time.
Understanding what is expected of them.
Getting homework and school notices to and from home/school efficiently.
Having the necessary "equipment" (lunch, musical instrument, PE kit, etc.) at school on the proper day.
Knowing how to interact socially or in a planned group activity: sharing, taking turns, feeling empathy (or even sympathy).
Being able to delay their need to do what they want to do when they want to do it.
Tolerating their own or others' mistakes.
Asking questions when they don't understand.
Planning and organizing their work.
Being consistent in their work, emotions, abilities and dependability.

Attention deficits and other learning styles are probably well enough understood today that most teachers realize they must present directions and instructions in a variety of ways so that visual, auditory, and kinaesthetic learners are all included. Teachers and instructors now know to break work assignments into smaller chunks for those who cannot process large quantities of materials all at one time. Good teachers are already utilizing these teaching techniques in their classroom, so they may wonder why they are still having difficulty managing the ADHD/ADD adopted/looked after child.

When considering the ADHD/ADD adopted/looked after child, there may be additionally complex issues that influence the behaviour of children in care. The latter children, very unintentionally, may be complicating the situation by virtue of their personal histories and backgrounds. It is not surprising that teachers would feel confused and perplexed by these children.

Following are some quite specific means of adapting a classroom to the needs of an adopted or looked after child who also manifests attention difficulties. Before the child is able to achieve the academic and behavioural performance the teacher, child, and parent/carer might be anticipating, the child is going to need to feel cared for, safe and structured at school. Perhaps some of the suggestions that follow will enable teachers to extrapolate their own ideas and strategies that will accommodate the particular ADHD/ADD adopted/looked after child in their classrooms.

When ADHD/ADD adopted/looked after children enter a classroom, they should know exactly what it is that they are supposed to do. It is best if "what they are supposed to do" is of high motivational interest. For example:

> Billy, who is an excellent artist and has a wonderful sense of humour, must be told that the moment he comes through the door, he should hang up his jacket, go to his desk, and start drawing a cartoon to share with his class at the opening of the class meeting. This gives Billy something to do that he is good at, that he likes to do, and that brings him positive attention from his classmates. At the same time, it keeps him out of the teacher's way, and apart from other children as everyone comes into the room. There is no extra work involved for the teacher in this scenario.
>
> Later in the day, when Billy has completed a short, but required amount of work, he might be allowed five minutes of time to either draw cartoons or to cut some out of magazines so that he will have them available to share with his classmates on mornings that he has trouble making up one of his own.

Virtually all children will have something they like to do that the teacher can adapt as a part of her repertoire of behaviour management techniques for a specific child. Almost always, these ideas can be used again, either as is, or almost as is, for another child, another time. Essentially, what the teacher wants to keep in mind is to devise an activity that will keep the child motivated and occupied in a productive manner and that enables the child to become a positive contributor to the classroom environment. It is also beneficial if the particular activity has room for expansion, remembering that the ADHD / ADD adopted / looked after child is going to be quickly and easily bored with repetition. In the case of Billy, he might begin to make a scrapbook of his cartoons and drawings or he might compile them in some way, for instance by subject matter, so he could pull out ones that he wanted when he wanted them.

There is a lot of social value in setting a task similar to the one above because it gives the ADHD / ADD adopted / looked after student an important role that may not have been possible otherwise. As these children often have trouble making friends, or behaving in a socially acceptable manner in school, giving them something to do that the rest of the class can enjoy or benefit from is tremendously valuable for them. In Billy's situation, he was so talented in his cartoon-making that it brought him many accolades from other students, and they were all eager to see each morning what he would produce.

There might be a child who is good at growing plants or one who is interested in recipes. Another child may have a particular interest in animals in general, or in one special animal. I once worked with a boy who was obsessed with Eurovision stars and songs, and another child who could tell me more about countries and flags than I had ever known previously. A young girl I knew loved making board games. All of these interests and many more can add significantly to any classroom at any level.

Like all children, ADHD / ADD adopted / looked after children learn best by doing, but these are children who really need to "do" in order to be able to stay focused on the task. This means that successful strategies for teachers to use are those that involve active participation. Having the chance to move around a lot is beneficial too. Maybe the child can lie down while reading in the library corner, stand while doing the art project, sit while writing and go to the blackboard now and again during maths. It seems strange, but many of these youngsters can listen better when the rest of their body is engaged. Doodling is a good thing, not a bad one. I even know children who listen best when they are playing a game or doing a puzzle.

Practitioners differ on this, but I am not convinced that these children listen more attentively when required to look at the person speaking. I have seen plenty of ADHD/ADD adopted/looked after children have no idea what the teacher said when it was demanded that the child look at the teacher. What can happen is that the child will focus on the spot of soup the teacher spilled on his shirt at lunch time, or the colour lipstick the teacher is wearing that reminds the child of a sister, or the tone of the teacher's voice which aggravates the student. Then, those distractions take the child off on a whole other train of thought, and they still have no idea of what the teacher said even though they appeared to be looking straight at her. It has been my experience that they often "hear" better if they can continue to engage in whatever it is they are already doing. It is important, however, to ask the child to repeat what the teacher (or parent/carer) just said because that is the only way the adult can really know if the child took in the information or not. (I would not want to deny that the child looking out the window may have been so intrigued by the orange butterfly that the child has absolutely no recollection at all of what the teacher's instructions were.) What the child subsequently does with the information may have no relevance to what he/she took in, but at least if one can be sure the child heard correctly what was said in the first place, it is a better start.

Another way to actively engage children in the classroom is by using the child's name frequently, but be sure this is only done in a positive way. We all pay attention to our own name, so using the child's name will bring him back in focus. The teacher can use the child's name when giving an example: if talking about action words or verbs, the teacher might say, "Nigel likes swimming." Perhaps the teacher could just add another bit to be sure that Nigel is really paying attention: "Nigel, you like to swim; what else do you like to do that is an action word?"

Having special chores in the classroom that require movement also help. This is the child who can run all of your errands for you, clean your blackboards, sharpen your pencils, hand out papers, empty the waste bins, or anything else you can think of that enables the child to get up and move about. As the teacher, you could even write your colleague upstairs a note and tell her that you just needed Austin to run an errand for you, so this note is serving that purpose. Put this in a sealed envelope because you can be sure that Austin is going to read any note that is in his hands. Giving an ADHD / ADD adopted / looked after child errands to run and jobs to do are not "rewards" for good behaviour; they are the means to the end, the way to acquire the behaviour you are looking for. These children need breaks and need activity and these are very legitimate ways of providing them with what they need. Moreover, the child often feels special to have been asked, and that adds to his / her feeling of trust and being trusted.

Another good job for these children might be the one of becoming the class "time monitor" for a week or so, alerting you to each time a half hour has passed—not that you particularly wanted or needed to know that, but if it keeps the child attentive, you'll be glad she told you. Many of these children are fascinated with timers of various sorts and often they get a bit fixated in "how long" something will take to do. Putting an egg-timer on the desk of a child and requiring him to do as many maths problems as he can before the timer finishes is a good way of keeping him focused and of motivating him to do a few more problems than maybe he would have done otherwise. The next day, the teacher could challenge the child to try to do one more problem than he'd done the day before. The teacher can also move the timer around the classroom so everyone has a chance to have it for a while. This should not be a competition; simply a means of helping those children who need to be more focused.

One more active idea for keeping ADHD / ADD adopted / looked after children attentive to what is going on in the lesson is by giving them a specific chore that has to do with the lesson. They could be asked to write the words on the board that the teacher is spelling or citing as important words. They can be given highlighters and asked to highlight specific words in their own reading material, such as all (or some) of the names of people or animals, or all of the verbs, or all of the words starting with a certain letter.

Many of these children do well having an activity book that they are allowed to work in when and if they accomplish what the teacher has asked them to do. For instance, if the student finishes writing out all of the spelling words, he should know that he can take out his word-search book and work in it until everyone in class is ready to move on to the next assignment or the teacher gives a new direction. Again, this is an activity that would benefit quite a few students in the classroom and that requires absolutely no extra energy from the teacher. It keeps distractible and/or very clever students from wasting time or getting themselves into trouble. When the ADHD/ADD adopted/looked after child is given something very specific to do, and when it is not too difficult for him/her to do what is being asked, it helps the child not only to focus on the work at hand, but also to be less susceptible to interfering emotional thoughts that may otherwise take up a substantial amount of the school day.

Keeping in touch

Teachers who can keep in touch frequently with students who have ADHD/ADD will find that the child is less likely to get off track, but "keeping in touch" does not necessarily mean in physical contact because, as has been said, children who have been abused may well not be receptive to hands-on. It is possible to touch the child's desk when you want to be sure that she is listening to important directions and it is possible to pay attention to the student personally as a means of being in touch. Simply asking the student, quietly, from time to time if everything is all right, may be one of the most valuable means of keeping the child more focused and on track. Similarly, as the teacher walks around the room, she can softly touch a corner of the desk or table where the distractible child is sitting. If, every once in a while, the teacher puts something on the desk, doing so will up the incentive for the child to pay attention. The teacher might just put down a sticker, an eraser, or pencil sharpener. Passing out happy faces will appeal to any young child in a classroom, and will help the unfocused child to pay attention when she sees the teacher walking by her desk.

Using unspoken signals generally works well. If the teacher can arrange a little conference with the student outside of classroom hours, they can set up signals that have meaning to them both. For example, if the teacher is in front of the class, he might hold up a ruler, which is the key for the ADHD/ADD adopted/looked after child to know that the next time the teacher asks a question, it will be asked of this child. That gives the child time to listen and prepare. The teacher must wait long enough to allow the child to have this composure time, but not so long that the child loses the train of thought. If the teacher is walking around the room, a certain number of fingers on the desk might tell the child that she is doing a good job at whatever it is that she is working on.

The child can give signals too. Often cards are used in these situations so that a child who is all of a sudden feeling unstable or worried can flash a card at the teacher which means the child needs to leave the room. When allowed to do this, most children will not "run". It is when they feel trapped and misunderstood that they run from classrooms and from school.

> Bennett was a great one for running until we introduced this system. It was made very clear to him that Mr Bay would allow him to leave the room when he really felt he needed to—and *before* he exploded—but that this privilege would be revoked if he left the school grounds. Bennett never once made any attempt to leave school after this system was instigated, and gradually his need to leave the classroom diminished, too.

Co-ordinating mental and physical attention through planned activities

With the current emphasis on whole body movement as a means of helping to rewire the brain synapses, and with the ADHD child's particular difficulty in staying in one position for an extended period of time, it is advantageous for teachers as well as parents/carers to think about strategies that might improve connections in the child's neurological structuring. As long ago as the 1960s, Jean Ayres (1973), was looking at the use of movement in helping children to feel more stabilized. In her work, she found that spinning some children on swings for a prescribed amount of time enabled them to work and feel better. Many occupational therapists today are utilizing these kinds of movement techniques when working with children who have a variety of physical and neurological deficits. Prescribed movements and pressures seem to be especially good for improving performance in activities such as handwriting, general co-ordination, concentration, and relaxation. Once more, however, some activities that are beneficial for children with attention disorders are not so good for children in care.

Generally speaking, it is not comfortable for children who have been abused to be involved with games that depend upon power struggles, such as tug-of-war, even though that push-pull activity does contribute to internal, physical pressure that works well for ADHD/ADD children. An alternative that can be used with both children is one that involves scarves or the kinds of bands used in Yoga with which one stretches and pulls against oneself.

Physical pressure is often used as a means of calming a child, but, at school in particular, it should not be someone else administering physical pressure on the child. It is the child who must create the physical pressure (as in doing push-ups on the floor or against a wall) that achieves the desired effect. Weight-bearing exercises are especially good, which is why teachers might want children to carry books or move chairs for them in the classroom.

Activities or games that involve lying on the floor or physically interacting with others (as in the game Twister or wheel-barrow races) are contra-indicated for many children in care.

Table 5 offers a few ideas that teachers might find useful for ADHD/ADD adopted/looked after children in the classroom and at school with regard to specific movements and activities that are fun and calming.

More and more frequently, psychologists/psychiatrists are also taking into account that neurology as well as psychology influences the child's thoughts and behaviours. As these professionals come to acknowledge that children from deprived or incompatible early experiences have neurobiological dysfunctions that need to be addressed in conjunction with, or even before, their emotional traumas, ADHD/ADD adopted/looked after children stand a better chance of becoming more successful adults (Cairns & Stanway, 2004; Lansdown, Burnell, & Allen, 2007; Silver, Amster, & Haecker, 1999).

Additional ideas and thoughts that may be useful

In the previous chapter, games that have an element of luck to them were mentioned as being useful methods of involving children in the learning process. Teachers can use Lady Luck in the classroom in many fun and creative ways, too. Remembering that it is not the

Table 5. Ideas for 2–5 minute movement breaks.

Things to do in the classroom
Assist teachers in carrying or shelving boxes, books and other "heavy" items.
Help to move chairs, tables, computers, or other furniture (being mindful of safety issues).
Take the register or notices to the office or to other classrooms.
Collect/distribute art materials or play equipment.
Sharpen pencils.
Hang things on or take things off of the bulletin board.
Take the waste bin around to collect rubbish from other students and from the floor.
All class activities that are good for everyone and particularly good for the ADHD/ADD adopted/looked after child
"Simon Says", but don't eliminate anyone.
Sit on chair with hands on either side of the seat. Raise self from the chair as many times as possible.
Rhythms or other hand-clapping games.
Individual or small group games: skipping ropes, hula hoops, jacks, hopscotch.
Relay races of all sorts, especially those that require attention, like keeping an egg or ball on the spoon.
Place hands on wall and do push-ups.
Cartwheels, headstands, gymnastics.

smartest person who wins the lottery numbers, it is the luckiest person, teachers can often engage recalcitrant or unfocused children in a variety of activities. Sometimes teachers have to "cheat" a little bit at luck, especially if they want to be sure that particular students stay with them throughout the game. Here is one way of doing this as part of a numbers lesson with young children.

You may be working on calendars or days and months of the year or on teaching children when their birthday is. If you are not sure that all of the children in your class actually do know when their birthday is, it is best to find out beforehand, and write down for each child on a separate piece of paper his/her date of birth.

Then you tell them that you have a game to play about birthdays and calendars and that the winner of the game will earn the chance to be the "change the calendar" person for the following week.

If you just want to leave luck to its own chances, you could say that all of the children who have a birthday in December should stand up. Then you could say if they have their birthday on a day with 2, 4, 6, or 8 in it, they should stay standing and everyone else sits down. This goes on until you select the particular number and one person wins.

On the other hand, if you are feeling the need for a particular child (like the ADHD or looked after child) to win because they have been having an especially good or bad day, then you would "cheat" and set up the game so that you previously select which birth date needs to win, and you eventually end the game with that "lucky" child coming out as the winner. If you are making the game work for a particular child, be sure you have chosen a reward for winning the game that actually has value to this child.

For older children, it is sometimes a good idea to reward the whole class when chance comes their way. Keeping lessons peppered with luck also keeps children more attentive. Maths games are especially good for this. Dice often work well. You could be looking at probability, but every time the total number eleven appears, everyone could earn a bonus point or a Smartie, etc. ADHD children are often very good at devising games, so you might occupy one of your more difficult students with the task of designing a game for you that has an element of chance as well as some elements of skill in it. Number games usually are objective enough so that children in care do not automatically have past associations with them and can thus stay focused without becoming so easily distracted.

> Jenny says, "When I sit in most of my classes, I keep thinking about things at home. I think about my dog, my sister, and my mother. I think about what I did last summer in the nice foster family and how much fun it would be to go back to see them this year. I think about next weekend and about having to see my dad in a Contact visit. I think about everything except school; but when we play those maths games it helps me to get away from all of this other thinking."

In line with having the whole class win something, I would refer back to Chapter Three, in which I suggest that all of the siblings earn a treat if they try to support their special needs brother or sister. I would recommend that teachers do something very similar, especially when trying to keep the ADHD/ADD adopted/looked after child from being bullied or wound-up. This is a child who is quite prone to bullying and to being bullied—a fact that all children in the classroom will have sussed out very quickly. To counteract this tendency, the teacher can set up points or rewards or incentives that will benefit the entire class rather than just one or two people.

For example, if Sally knows that she never can answer enough geography questions to come out on top, and if Mark feels that he is such a poor speller that he will be spelled-out in the first round, either or both of these children might find it amusing to tease or annoy Jared because they know he is in foster care and that he cries easily. Sally might begin to tease him about forgetting so much stuff that he probably forgot where he left his mother, and Mark tells Jared that he's stupid because he can't even read a comic book properly.

However, if the teacher has set up the incentive that the whole class can win a homework-free night if, as a class, they earn up to seventy-five points for everyone's total correct answers, then children like Sally and Mark are going to try harder themselves, and they are more likely to help Jared come up with the right answer (they might even cheat and tell him the right answer!) because it is to everyone's advantage for all of them collectively to earn a lot of points.

Such an incentive produces many good end results: each child tries harder, each child tries to help the other children, and children like Jared are supported by their classmates rather than teased by them. Once again, this does not take any extra time or work on the teacher's part, and it adds considerably to a day well spent in the classroom. If the children do earn the homework-free night, it even lightens the teacher's load because there is then no homework to have to mark!

If one has accepted the fact that rewarding individuals is a good thing to do, then the use of incentives and reinforcements in the classroom will go a very long way. If an ADHD/ADD adopted/looked after child always has a difficult time in the lunch queue or in the dining hall, it makes sense to partner that child with someone for whom these are not overwhelming tasks. The important part is to rotate who the partner is so that no child feels burdened by having to be the "assistant", but at the same time, each child can feel that he/she is making a positive contribution to another classmate by helping out. If the teacher either needs to lean on one child for a bit, or if there is a child who voluntarily is outstandingly helpful, it is my view that that person should be acknowledged quietly, perhaps a bit behind the scenes, with an extra "treat". This treat can take the form of a certain privilege that the teacher knows is meaningful to the helping person. (If the teacher makes a big deal of this in front of the class however, the child will soon be singled out as "teacher's pet," so it is a good idea to keep it quiet.)

ADHD/ADD adopted/looked after children almost always do need help on the playground. That is, generally speaking, one of the hardest parts of their school day because there is no structure and no pattern that they can anticipate or follow. Their impulsivity and immediate need for gratification tend to get them into squabbles and difficulties from the word go. If they want the ball, they are likely to take it—and not give it back. Sharing is often an impossible task. Joining a game nicely rarely works for them. If they are accidentally bumped into, they perceive it as a major attack, and one that requires retaliation. If children are laughing, this child will construe that they are laughing at her. Alternatively, the ADHD/ADD adopted/looked after child will sit alone, play by himself, and feel completely isolated with no one to call a friend.

Although the management of children who need social support at home and at school is discussed in the subsequent chapter, a small suggestion for teachers who know that play time is difficult for one of their children is to try to involve the dinner lady or another child in giving the ADHD/ADD adopted/looked after child something specific to do on the playground. The dinner lady might ask this child to guess with her how many children each of them thinks is wearing a red shirt that day (or a bow in their hair if school uniforms are worn). After each has guessed, the child could go around the playground and count the number of red shirts or bows. Similarly, one child could be specifically asked to include the ADHD/ADD adopted/looked after child in their game of rounders. The teacher also can give the child a playground "job" to do such as measuring the space between the school building and the school fence with the tape measure that the teacher loans to the child. Subsequently, the teacher can use that measurement information in a project or activity.

Conclusion

As has been pointed out, there are shelves and shelves of books in libraries and bookshops that address behaviour management strategies for children with attention difficulties, and there are equal numbers that tell teachers how to set up the classroom and teach the child with ADHD / ADD. Virtually all of these books have many good strategies and very important suggestions, most of which usually have quite a positive effect.

There are far fewer books of a similar nature that suggest how to manage adopted and looked after children, although, increasingly, there are publications that deal with the specific issues of abuse and neglect and there are several good "how-to" books written by counsellors in group homes that deal with behaviour management for foster carers.

All of this literature provides a useful and important read, and one will learn many new strategies in the reading. The downside of these books, though, is that they often purport to solve all of your problems and to provide answers to all of your dilemmas. Whether teacher, parent, or carer, you could be disappointed if you do what the book tells you to do and "it still doesn't work". You also might begin to feel pretty awful about yourself if you cannot make it work when the book almost guarantees that if you do it right, the results will be on your doorstep.

In my own experience, you can line up all of the dominoes exactly right and there can still be an ill wind that keeps them from falling down in the perfect synchronicity that you sought. People just do not always do things the way we want them to or think that they should.

Maybe you, as a teacher, think you have taught six times seven in all of the kinaesthetic, auditory, visual, and creative ways you have been taught to do, but, for whatever reason, Ali still cannot remember that six times seven is forty-two. Then, all of a sudden, Ali comes to school one day and tells you he knows forever after that six times seven is forty-two. "How do you know that, Ali?" you ask, with awe. "Because my father is forty-two and he has six moles on one arm and seven on the other," he replies with assurance.

Well, that was a strategy that you were not very likely to hit upon, and it certainly was not going to be found in one of those books on your shelf; but sure enough, it worked for Ali!

The more methods of teaching, of managing behaviour, and of learning that we can take on board, the better strategists each of us will become (Weaver, 1994). We need to have a bottomless bag to which we can keep adding strategies at the same time that we reach inside to pull out what we think might be best for the child who is puzzling us or who is sitting in the front row of our classroom. Yes, most ADHD/ADD children respond to structure and consistency and predictability, and usually, to the extent that you provide all of these, the child will adapt more readily. Similarly, most adopted/looked after children walk into your classroom with a background that may defy your worst nightmares, and so they need safety and calmness and understanding, as well as a much better education than they have probably had in the past. The combination of ADHD/ADD and adoption/fostering can be lethal, or it can be a challenge to a teacher's creativity and sensitivity.

In one teacher's room, I saw written on the blackboard:

> "What part of 'quiet' did you not understand?"

I am not sure whether this is unnecessary sarcasm or a legitimate means for the teacher to try to inject some humour and relate to her students. It points out why our efforts to be creative must also be sensitive.

This chapter is full of thoughts and strategies that can only serve as ideas and suggestions, because none of them is either infallible or comprehensive. At best, they will offer a point of departure and they may help when your own engine is falling off the tracks. More importantly, the chapter requests that all of us make a big effort to look deeply into the hearts and souls of the children who sit in front of us trying their hardest to learn while their thoughts and feelings are guiding them elsewhere. It is so easy to feel angry with these children, but their own anger and hurt is far more seething and painful than is ours. Trying to work out how to get past this valley of despair, whether it comes from a mind that does not do what you want it to do when you want it to, or from a life of hunger and emptiness, or both, will bring out empathy and a sense of accomplishment in both the teacher and the child.

CHAPTER FIVE

Social development in the ADHD/ADD adopted/ looked after child

Daniel engages easily with adults, much more so than with peers, and enjoys one-to-one attention with an adult who shows interest in him. At six years old, he still prefers to play with the toys in his own way and without anyone else joining in. If another child comes near him, it makes him lose his concentration and he becomes irritable.

"I've only had toys since I was adopted," he says. "It's too hard to share them, and I can't stand it if anyone else changes my stuff around. If I set something up, it has to be up to me, not anyone else, to decide whether it gets moved or not . . . it makes me too mad when it can't be my way."

Like a much younger child, Daniel "needs" to determine the rules of the game and he "has" to play with toys when and how he wants them to be played with. His dad says that he intellectually understands this, but it keeps him from being able to spend quality time with Daniel because there is so little interaction possible.

* * *

Christie, still in a foster home, doesn't have anything to play with that she can call her own. "I tend not to play too much with other kids' stuff," she says, "because I don't want to get blamed for it if something

> gets broken. I stay to myself and don't mess with the other kids because I feel safer that way.
>
> "It would be nice to have friends, I guess; but either I move or they move and I don't really know what to talk to girls about anyway. I think all of us in this house keep a lot of secrets, and at school, it's scary because you don't want to say something that you're going to be sorry about later. People can turn on you, so it's best to stay quiet and to yourself."

ADHD/ADD adopted/looked after children are often particularly vulnerable to social developmental disorders. Neither their early experiences nor their attention difficulties contribute to positive or age appropriate social interactions. Moreover, a 1996 research study on antisocial behaviour that used an adoption design (Ge, et al., 1996), found that when biological parents had substance abuse problems or antisocial personality disorder, the adopted children were much more likely to be hostile and antisocial than were adoptees from untroubled biological parents (p. 42). This inherited tendency was manifested by being temperamental, having problems with emotional self-control, acting impulsively, and exhibiting attention dysfunctions. Infants and young children who present with early personality and character difficulties, as we have seen, usually evoke more severe responses from their care-takers, which, of course, in turn, exacerbates the antisocial behaviour.

Given the possibilities of a disposition to antisocial behaviour, and since ADHD/ADD adopted/looked after children easily misconstrue what they see and hear, these children tend to lack social coherence in their lives, and thereby often have trouble constructing a meaningful context for themselves in the world around them. This is especially true for the children in the care system who have experienced multiple moves, many of which could have happened without much or any prior warning. A lack of social coherence and meaning also shows up among children whose relationships with others depended upon sex, goods, favours, or adult, rather than child, needs.

As ADHD/ADD adopted/looked after children often are still struggling to come to terms with their own emotional and physiological cues, it is easy to understand why they may not be able to tune into the emotions and concerns of others. Although many adopted and looked after youngsters are extremely street-savvy and are unusually aware of and attentive to the nuances of sounds and movements of a chaotic environment, their wisdom and selective attention are rather circumscribed, and usually not in synchrony with the families who take them in. The behaviour that the child brings into the new home or school makes sense to the child, but, for the most part, this child has previously learnt an unhelpful script for the environment into which he/she is being placed.

In some or many respects, the child's language and actions might not be relevant to, or acceptable in, mainstream family living. A child who has been exposed to a violent atmosphere might have very rude language at ready command. The impulsivity, if this is a child with ADHD/ADD, will mean that there is rarely a check point at which use of language will be self-monitored, even after the child has been told that those words are not allowed in the home or school. Aggressive behaviour is commonly observed in both ADHD children and in children who are or have been in the care system. This is spontaneous, defensive behaviour, and it is not easy to diminish the ingrained, reflexive responses to stimuli that are perceived as being threatening.

For a looked after child who has had multiple placements, entering a new house is similar to what most of us would experience in moving from country to country when many of the customs and mores of each country differ. Perhaps we have just learnt to delicately balance the shrimp on the chopsticks when we are then thrust into a home where food is eaten only with hands—but, actually, only with the right hand. In these situations, we would have to do a lot of observing and guessing and asking. Probably, we would tend to make many mistakes. After so much travel, we are usually tired, and want to "go home". This is what the child in care would like to do, too, only there is no going home for so many of these youngsters.

Children who are adopted from overseas have even greater barriers to cross than those who have been in just one country. A longitudinal study of children adopted internationally who were receiving classroom accommodation or special education found that the most common diagnosis of problematic behaviour was ADHD/ADD, occurring in 25% of the children (primarily in boys) (Glennen & Bright, 2005). Behaviour profiles in this study indicated higher than average levels of hyperactivity, and that the child's expressive vocabulary at 2–3 years of age predicted his/her outcomes for social skills and problem behaviours.

Although many foreign-adopted children leave their native homeland before they have actual speech, that child will still have been exposed to the sounds of the native language. Similarly, the sights and smells of the child's environment, even if it were just an orphanage or institutional environment, will be unique to the country and the care-taking individuals of that country. Adjusting to a whole new world is not easy for any child, especially not a child whose attachments are already fragile and who is leaving an environment that is familiar, even if not pleasant. All or any of these children might easily present with many similar characteristics to ADHD/ADD children who have not yet acquired the social mores of their peers. Extra time, understanding, and support, as well as additional social instruction, are often needed for children adopted from abroad.

> Monihito came to England from Japan when he was eight years old—quite old for a foreign-adopted child, but his adoptive parents were British, living in Japan when they adopted him. As he went to Japanese schools in Tokyo, his behaviour at school was guided by Japanese customs. His teacher in England was often annoyed with Monihito because he would never look at her when she spoke to him. In Japan, however, it is rude for a child to look at an adult, so Monihito always politely bowed his head and lowered his eyes when spoken to.

All children who have come into care, not just internationally adopted children, will experience a certain amount of language and sensory organization disruption. It is as though they are strung to a different scale, because, as we have seen, the sensory environment in one's early months plays an important part in the development of the growing brain and in the emotions of the child. Like the instrument that is out of tune with the rest of the orchestra, this musical member could be at odds with what is being played around him.

The subtleties of verbal and body language may not be obvious to a child moving into a new situation. Adopted/looked after children have had to make many adjustments in their young lives in order to try to accommodate themselves to others, although being short on attention and long on distractibility, some of these children may never have paid much attention to those cues that could have been helpful to improving their social relationships. Moreover, if something like acquiring enough food, or holding on to a certain possession, or making sure no one is lurking around behind you, is what is constantly on your mind, you may easily become overly focused on self-protection, and not have much time to think about social "niceties" anyway. It is very probable that good manners have not been of great importance in the lives of children who are struggling to stay alive and safe or to children who cannot even focus on the basic and fundamental aspects of home and school living, let alone on being polite.

When children, figuratively, have gone to the same film but have seen and heard a different sound-track from either the adult who went with them or other children who saw the same movie, it can be extremely confusing for both parties. In this same sense, it is not unusual for children who have been traumatized to perceive their surroundings askew from the way other people see them, and then, of course, they respond to their own perceptions, as we all do. Other times they may see the event similarly, but their reaction to it becomes grossly out of proportion to the reality.

If I am driving down the street and see that a police car is behind me, I will check to see that I am within the speed limit and will have a brief review of other related issues, such as if my registration plates are in order. Then I am likely to let go of the situation and carry on with the police car behind me.

The traumatized individual, however, may be in the same situation and go into a panic that the police car is not merely "behind" but is "following" him. He may lose his ability to think rationally, and will ignite a long-ago memory that associated the police with violence and disruption in his childhood. This reminiscence could lead the driver to become careless on the road, at which point, sure enough, the police car will pull him over, and a confrontation will occur. As such, the saga goes on of one small innocuous incident culminating in an aggressive, exaggerated, irrational (by other peoples' standards) and debilitating event.

In their own ways and within the context of their own stories, this is what can happen to ADHD / ADD adopted / looked after children, too. It is usually why other children don't like to play with them or be with them—because their behaviour is too unpredictable and because they get "mad" too easily.

> Joyce doesn't want to come outside with her bat and ball if Simon is around because Simon will grab the bat and start hitting other people or things with it. It is not a lot of fun for her to try to be Simon's friend.
>
> Having the bat in his own hand rather than in someone else's may be Simon's way of feeling that he is in control and safe, but it is not the way his neighbours and classmates operate.

One observes children who misperceive spoken communication just as easily as they do non-verbal situations. What is confusing is that the child may actually hear and understand individual words, but getting the meaning of these words all together is an arduous task. Sometimes the child understands all of the words, and may even remember them verbatim; yet, the child does not actually appreciate the gist of what is being said. It is quite possible to repeat a series of words that have no coherent meaning even when one knows the meaning of the individual words: "Today dinner for want you do what," does not make sense to me, although I do know each of those words by itself. When something does not come across coherently, we try to remember or latch on to a part of what was said and then we respond to that piece of the whole. In this case, the child with an attention difficulty might focus on the word "today" because it was the first word in the sentence, and the child would then reply to something in his head that had to do with "today". The adopted/looked after child, on the other hand, might respond to the word "dinner" since dinner is something that child never had enough of. This child could also reply inappropriately, as in, "The teacher makes me stay inside at dinnertime." In an earlier chapter, Daniel experienced his social worker telling him that he needed to get "adjusted" before he could see his sister. Daniel understood the meaning of "adjust" when applied to "adjusting your chair so you can sit more comfortably at the table", but he was unable to make sense of "adjust" in the social worker's terminology and context.

Miscommunication may be why teachers and parents/carers frequently complain that children are not listening or that they are being cheeky or rude in their replies. Indeed, they may be; but also, they may not have accurately perceived the message, whether visually or auditorily. Not just ADHD/ADD or adopted/looked after children do this. Other youngsters with various processing disorders get things muddled up, too. In general, many disorganized children might have trouble reading the social cues that others take for granted. Most youngsters do not have much patience with this kind of behaviour when it happens repeatedly, especially if no one has explained to them why a child is behaving the way he is. Not infrequently, other children either avoid the child who acts differently or belligerently, or they make them targets for bullying.

A place to play

Communication skills are vitally important with regard to having friends and making good social adjustments. Many communication skills, whether verbal or non-verbal, are learned by young children through play; yet, play time seems to have been significantly absent in the lives of almost all children in the care system. In the normal course of growing up, most children will be at the park, or in the home of another child, or at a church or social function where they will stand and watch other children, play next to another child, or engage in play with another child or children. In this way they learn what is "socially acceptable" and what is not, and they develop and practise their own skills in the process.

Social and emotional development can be seriously injured if a child is deprived of opportunities to play and interact with others. It has already been stressed in this book that a child needs to have a sensitive and attentive care-giver who can stimulate the child through growth-producing activities; but it is equally important for a baby and toddler to have some chances to interact with other children. Playing is how babies engage others in their lives, and how they begin to understand their world. Spontaneously, infants will use all of their senses and all of their body when they start to play. Within the first nine months of life, a child will have acquired a phenomenal amount of information just from playing. For most infants, their parents and siblings take delight in playing with them, which is what makes this interactive process so positive.

Sadly, children in the care system have not had this experience and have missed out on some very important learning lessons. The results of lack of stimulation or inappropriate stimulation in playful activities will be reflected in the child's neurological and social development. For the baby who consistently does not receive positive reinforcement for eliciting attention from an adult, play will not become integrated as a pleasurable, reciprocal and valuable activity. The lack of play can impair a child's ability to focus, to think imaginatively and to respond with sensitivity. Play should be a "problem-solving" activity for the young child, but the absence of play deprives children of a normal and natural means of working out how to negotiate difficult situations or to express feelings.

On the flip side of that same coin, children with attention deficits are hard for others to play with. Even very patient parents/carers will become exasperated with a child who flits from one activity to another, and who cannot focus on anything long enough to have meaningful interaction with the toy or book or puzzle or person, and who has to have everything done in his/her own way. Indeed, these are not fun children with whom to play, and so the cycle of frustration on both sides intensifies.

When a child does not have a chance to learn how to play, the child will not be able to learn from playing. Many looked after children arrive in care having already turned inside themselves and cannot play with others, or do not want others to play with them. These children usually display an extremely short attention span when given the opportunity to play in their new home, because they may not know how to interact with a toy in order to make it come alive for them. They usually choose toys of a much younger developmental and age level than their own chronological age, and they rarely want anyone else to be involved in their play.

As they have had so few experiences playing by themselves and/or with other babies, looked after children usually have received little chance or encouragement to develop and practise the social and thinking skills they need in order to be prepared for getting along in the world. Children who know how to make friends are practising their skills every day, but most of the skills they practise are already fairly proficient. What they are doing is fine-tuning the basics. For children who have poor adult models, few or no child companions, lives of abuse and neglect, and experiences of violence or abandonment, there is a lack of knowledge base for much of anything relating to playful times. These children need to be taught socially acceptable means of interrelating so that they can acquire, and then practise, new and more beneficial ways of interacting.

Nobody wants to be my friend

Unfortunately, the impulsivity and lack of empathy afflicting large numbers of ADHD/ADD adopted/looked after children impedes their ability to make and keep the friendships they so desperately need to have. Although adults may be concerned about the child's inability to achieve academic success at school, most young children will be far less bothered by poor marks than they will be by poor social relationships. Knowing that you will be the last one chosen for anything, that no one wants to be your partner, that the seat next to you on the school bus is always going to be empty, and believing that you were not even good enough for your mother to want you or take care of you, is not a nice way to wake up in the morning. Sadly, however, the repertoire of defences that this child wears as a suit of armour is not easily broken into, so the carousel often goes around and around with a disappointing stagnancy. Even very sensitive parents/carers and extremely patient teachers are often not enough to interrupt such a cycle once it has become well established. Friendless children who are unusually despondent, angry, alone, and aggressive generally are those who would benefit from seeing a therapist—again, one who understands and values the unique medical and social history that this child brings to the table.

The skills children learn through their friendships with peers are skills that they will retain throughout their lives, with successful relationships greatly influencing a child's self-esteem. Richard Lavoie (2006) points out that positive relationships with peers are known to have a significant effect on a child's sense of self and on his/her well-being. "Professionals have come to realize the critical fact that a child's social life—often referred to as 'the other sixteen hours'—is immeasurably important to his happiness, health and development" (p. xxv).

Remembering that ADHD/ADD adopted/looked after children already have a physiological make-up that is more geared towards self-preservation and that is highly attuned to danger, it is important to appreciate the neurobiological factors that can influence their relationships with others. From primitive man onwards, the fight/flight response was programmed into people in order to protect them from environmental dangers. Just like the caveman who faces the hungry lion, the child who is familiar with trauma will react with whatever emotion seems appropriate to him in a situation that he deems frightening. Since much that goes on positively in a child's daily environment can be easily misconstrued by the child who has only experienced negativity, this child may well perceive everyday actions from other adults and children as being aggressive or scary behaviours from which he must protect himself.

> Melissa, a child with significant attention and emotional difficulties, is seven years old and in foster care. Her early life of deprivation and abandonment have reinforced her belief that she is not ever going to be given anything nice and that nothing ever belongs to her. Melissa is out on the school playground when Diane arrives at school and joins her friends to play catch with the new purple ball the class has just been given. Melissa wants that purple ball, and she wants to play with the other girls, but she does not know how to ask or to join the game. When Diane misses the ball and it rolls by Melissa, she picks it up and runs away with it. Diane calls to her to give it back, but Melissa pays no attention. Now, all of the girls run towards Melissa, who gets scared and puts her school pencil into the ball, popping and ruining it. From Melissa's viewpoint, of course she cannot now give the ball back because she does not have the ball, and it was not her fault for breaking it because they were chasing her and were going to hurt her.

This was clearly a no-win situation, but while the other girls now do not have a ball to play with, poor Melissa has neither a ball nor a friend. In fact, she has dug her hole even deeper, because none of the girls in that group wants to be her friend.

Initially, there was no real danger for this little girl, but her perception of the potential for something to go wrong was heightened when she realized that the other girls had something she didn't, and that she had no way of getting. As the ball came to her, her impulsivity and her intense need to have something for herself created stress, anxiety, and a perceived danger, so she ran. Then the danger did become real because all of the girls were chasing after her. This situation grew well out of proportion to what could have happened had Melissa simply been able to pick up the ball and throw it back to the girls, who might even have invited her to play with them. The exaggerated response stemmed from Melissa's internal needs and her inability to control herself in the situation. Since there was not an adult present to mediate the interactions so that it would have had a more positive outcome for Melissa, this single experience will be added to her previous catalogue of sorrows about no one wanting to be her friend.

Most children do not like to be different from their peers. Thus, they will do everything they can to be and to do the same as everyone else, but only in so far as that behaviour feels self-preserving or rewarding for them. When they cannot, or feel that they cannot, keep up with their peers, they might begin to withdraw or to act out rather atrociously. Some elect to become the class clown, a tactic that often draws a lot of peer support, especially among boys. Others behave outrageously, perhaps in the hope of being excluded from school—a perceived safer option than staying in school where they are failing so miserably. Some just try to meet their own needs in whatever way they can, whether it is by disassociating themselves or by becoming very aggressive. Alexander is a good example of how enormously disruptive children can be helped to have better relationships at school and in their later lives.

> Alexander, a thirteen-year-old who lived back and forth between his grandmother's house and a foster carer's home, was a young man with a bookshelf full of difficulties. What I felt to be quite a dramatic "case" of ADHD, the medical professionals involved consistently denied, putting his extreme behaviour down to emotional problems—of which there were many, I was the first to acknowledge.
>
> Alexander was the absolute prototype of a child who persistently felt the need to get himself excluded from school—a position that was remarkably easy for him to achieve, despite the fact that he was already in a special school for "emotionally–behaviourally disturbed" children. He was a child who knew well how to get out of school, both literally and figuratively. Alexander would run, throw chairs, curse teachers, threaten and fight students. These behaviours quickly bought him a ticket home, which is where he preferred to be. Not only did he feel safer at home (at his grandmother's house), but also he felt the need to be there for her, as she was not well.

I knew Alexander and worked with him for quite a few years. In the course of that time, I never doubted that his familial situation caused enormous emotional problems for him, but I also felt that what I considered to be his severe ADHD was also interfering with his ability to improve. Although Alexander was never hostile or violent in our Centre, he was always the classic ADHD child, meriting almost all of the ticks on the ADHD criteria list.

Subsequent to a very long struggle, Alexander was finally put on medication at the same time that his grandmother, the foster carer, the school, and I worked out some intense school and home adjustments to meet his needs. One important adjustment the school nicely agreed to was allowing Alexander to carry his cell phone so he could ring his grandmother when he became anxious about her or about himself. This worked a miracle, and was a significant factor in helping Alexander to get along throughout the school day.

Alexander had (still has) an absolute fetish with the Rolling Stones. As his behaviour settled, he was able to share this interest with two other classmates, and the three of them eventually produced a play that was put on for the entire school, bringing the boys "fame and glory".

Today, at twenty-one, Alexander holds a job in a grocery store, maintains a few friendships—maybe "acquaintenance-ships" is a better definition—with his workmates, and continues to listen to the Stones. He and his grandmother are still doing well together.

"I just know"

If one watches children at a public park or on the school playground, it is fascinating to note that the vast majority of youngsters are able to anticipate what happens in social situations. They absorb this information with amazing speed, alacrity, and accuracy. They are also able to interpret other children's reactions and moods so that they know who is angry or annoyed, and they know, too, when someone is pleased or happy. Even very young toddlers soon learn to read body language and other non-verbal communication as well as the spoken word—sometimes better than the spoken word. In addition, these children have a certain know-how and ability to adjust their own behaviours to those of others. Children who do this without undue effort figure out that there is a give and take in conversations and in play long before they ever enter school. If older children are asked how they know how to do these things, they usually have no specific answer: they "just know".

Significant numbers of children with various learning and living disorders do not "just know". The unwritten rules for establishing and maintaining friendships remain a mystery to them. For many ADHD/ADD adopted/looked after children, who may well fall into the group of youngsters who do not "just know", the nature of their attention disorder and the circumstances of their early lives drive away the very people who potentially would mean the most to them. Their attitudes and behaviours make them out of step with their peers as well as with the adults who are responsible for them even though friends and family are what they most crave.

Despite the fact that there is an enormous amount of technology to help those children who have minor or even very severe physical or learning difficulties, there is as yet no machine or programme that enables a child to read social cues or to make a friend. This may be why so many people turn to chat lines on the Internet, because it is a way of communicating with others that is less affected by incompetent social skills and there is no body language to interpret. One can take a break from the conversation by walking away from the computer, or one can discontinue the interaction temporarily and resume later with no significant disruption. This is not possible when two people are together in the same space.

Some helpful intervention ideas and strategies

On the other hand, there are therapeutic interventions that can be very successful, and even parents and carers can practise many of these techniques at home with their children (Webster-Stratton, 1999). A young child's board game called "Look Before You Leap" is a game of frogs that encourages children to do just what the game is called—look before leaping. When children can learn to curb some of their impulsivity, they work more effectively with others in groups or in pairs. There are also games that require players to match up words or phrases with the look on a person's face (picture cards with faces on them). Other games involve one player listening while the other player describes a wish or feeling or experience, and then they trade positions.

I am an advocate of using pre-school storybooks for a wide range of ages when children need to learn about friendship skills. *Frog and Toad are Friends* (Lobell, 1979), *Best Friends for Frances* (Hoban, 1969), *George and Martha* (Marshall, 1972), and *No Fighting, No Biting!* (Minarik, 1958) are among my personal favourites for looking at how others think about and make friends, but any book that the reader enjoys is a good one to share with a child. These kinds of books can lead to many good discussions and thoughts about what are some good ways of making and being a friend. Parents and carers do not need any professional skills for reading storybooks with children. As a matter of fact, they do not even really need to know how to read, because there are many beautiful picture books without words that the adult and child can look at to create their own meanings.

Sometimes the parent/carer and child can make up their own book by drawing a picture of whatever they want (or one pertaining to a particular topic, such as "rain" or "a birthday party") and then they can write a story about it, or just talk about it. If wanting to work on friendship skills, it is a good idea for the adult to think of a rather open subject to draw, but one that could include some aspect of friendship. Even if the child does not draw a relevant picture, the adult could do so, and then they could talk about it together with the following kind of conversation.

Adult draws a sad child.

Adult:	Why is she sad?
Child:	Because she didn't get invited to the birthday party.
Adult:	Why might that be?
Child:	Because no one wants to play with her.
Adult:	How could she act differently so that next time someone might want to invite her?

Another way of using stories and pictures is to draw or look at pictures that have no captions. Then the adult and child can make up captions or can draw bubbles over people's heads and write a conversation into the bubbles. It is important in all of these instances to let the child draw, write, and say whatever he/she wants to. Their statements will tell the adult something about how the child is thinking, and the children need to know that whatever they say is going to be acceptable.

> Taylor, an adopted eight-year-old, was playing with Play Dough in the art room with the classroom aide he has because of his attention difficulties. Taylor repetitively made "poop sandwiches" and offered them to the aide.
>
> "Yuck, Taylor, you don't want to make those; don't make those sandwiches, Taylor. That's not nice."
>
> Taylor did want to make poop sandwiches though, and insisted on doing so. After watching these interactions for a while, I sat down with Taylor and the aide, and asked Taylor what he was making.
>
> "Poop sandwiches."
>
> "Oh."
>
> "Do you want one?"
>
> "Well, I don't really like poop sandwiches, so I'll pass. Did you have one yourself?"
>
> "Not now, but before I did."

This was an important piece of Taylor's background that he was trying to tell others about, and an issue that certainly needed to be talked about with him. Children's play and stories are the ways they know to talk about and tell about what is of interest or concern to them.

Another word to say about books and stories is that it is extremely helpful if parents and carers can help their children to know what other children are reading so the child can join in on those conversations. Pre-school children like nursery rhymes and fairy tales. The child in care probably never had a book read to him/her, so teaching these stories can help them to keep up with their peers. Similarly, with older children, it is good to help your child read whatever typical book or fad-book other peers are reading at the moment. If the book is too difficult for your child to read on his own, you can read it to him.

Teachers in school do well to spend time once in a while talking with groups of children about social skills and friendships. Relatively generalized conversations revolving around such topics as: "What do we mean by 'friendship'?", or "What do you value most in a friend?" are good ways to elicit various students' thoughts and ideas about what they expect from a friend and how they feel they need to contribute to the relationship. The ADHD/ADD adopted/looked after child may have much to gain by hearing what others say. As we all know, there is nothing more effective than learning from peers, especially when it is in a calm and controlled setting. These class conversations are equally as important in secondary school as they are in the younger years.

A common difficulty for children who lack social skills is that they do not know how to join a group. Many impulsive children, or those youngsters who are typically left on the outside of groups, really have little idea of how it is that others manage to be a part of a game or a circle of friends. Even when teachers put children together for a project, the ADHD/ADD adopted/looked after child may not understand the dynamics of group activity—like taking your turn, being patient, sharing, not dominating, etc.

Younger children might be taught to think about how groups work and how one joins in when wanting to play with a group of kids who are already involved in an activity together:

- watch the group for a little while if you want to join it;
- try to find someone you know who is playing, or someone who seems as if he/she might be kind if you asked to join;
- don't ask the whole group, but find the one person from above, and ask that person if you could play too;
- (schools should not allow children to say "You can't play!");
- if someone says "No", try to smile and wait until another time;
- if someone says: "Wait a minute", do try to wait a bit, and then ask again if no one has included you. (Waiting is not easy for ADHD children.)
- as a last resort, ask a teacher if she can help you to join the group. (It is a last resort because the other children probably will not like it that the child told on them for not letting the child play.)

With older children, role-playing and acting in skits are often a valuable means of learning about and teaching group-joining skills. It is also very beneficial for all students to think about how and when to invite others to join in their games or conversations. It is amazing how little effort it takes to ask another: "Do you want to play?" Five small words can make all of the difference in the world to a child who has never, ever been asked this before.

Schools should consider having play policies that resist a "You can't play" attitude. Playgrounds need to be better staffed and monitored so that children are not allowed to be excluded from games. Adopted / looked after children, while being extremely vulnerable to being bullied, also know how to be major bulliers themselves. These children, especially those who also act impulsively and aggressively, need assistants on the playground (and in the changing rooms) so as to minimize the possibilities of bullying incidents.

When helping children with peer relationships, it is useful to have them think about their own behaviours, and then to wonder with them if they think other children would agree or disagree with the way they describe themselves. This could be a scary task for ADHD / ADD adopted / looked after children, so care must be taken that they do not feel threatened or exposed during this kind of exercise. It is definitely not a group exercise, but one to be worked on with a parent / carer or individually with a teacher or therapist.

There are times when the adult in charge will be astonished at the way a particular child is acting because it seems so inappropriate for the situation at hand. In these instances, it can be good to ask that child what she thinks is happening, so that you have a better perspective of what she might be feeling or experiencing that is contrary to or different from what you are anticipating or observing. In these instances, I might tell a child that it is all right if he sees a situation in a certain way, but I think it would be helpful for him to know that MOST other people see the same situation differently, and then explain to the child how most other people would interpret the situation.

Laura is ten years old and was adopted five years ago. She had been in a foster family who lived near the mountains, where the family often spent snowy weekends. Laura was very fond of the foster family and loved their times together in the snow. She now lives in a warm, urban area with the family who adopted her.

In an unusual winter that was exceptionally cold, Laura's PE teacher brought enormous wheelbarrows full of snow to the school playground

> and dumped them out for all the children in the class to play in. Laura, however, became oblivious to everyone else. Upon seeing and feeling the snow, she remembered back to the early days of her life near the mountains. Laura lay down, spread-eagled in the snow; she gathered up huge quantities of the snow and began to build her own snowman and igloos, not allowing anyone else near her. Her exuberance in her prior happy memory had completely overtaken her.
>
> When the PE teacher talked to Laura about what was going on, Laura said that she thought the snow was brought for her and that she could play however she wanted to in it. Laura's intensity to gratify her own needs obscured her ability to grasp that this was a group activity and that she was required to share. Even with considerable input from the very kind PE teacher, Laura had great difficulty understanding or empathizing with the fact that other children also wanted to play with the snow, and that it was for all of them to do together.

These are just a few of the kinds of behaviours that get in the way of friendship-making. For some children, they may only occur periodically, and therefore, these children may have some ability to make and retain a friend or two. For other children, the skills required for making and being a friend remain elusive. In the same way that the luckiest, not the smartest, person wins the lottery, the "nicest", rather than the most intelligent, person tends to have more friends, although certainly this can be one and the same person at times. ADHD/ADD adopted/looked after children may need considerable input to learn the social skills that come more naturally to others, and they definitely will need to be given many, many opportunities to practise and hone their newly acquired "niceties".

Self-esteem and self-confidence

Children whose developmental histories keep them at risk for social and educational difficulties are frequently the same children who experience low self-esteem. Sometimes, as in the earlier example of Billy, the cartoonist, a child's difficulties can be overridden by an outstanding talent, especially if it happens to be a talent that other children value. In such instances, the child's feeling of self-worth might be slightly enhanced, and the "Nobody likes me"; "Nobody will play with me"; "I can't do anything right" feelings could be less pervasive than for those children who do not have a special talent to fall back on.

Feeling good about oneself, however, certainly does not need to be the result of having an extraordinary talent. In fact, most of us probably do not have truly outstanding aptitudes; but we tend to feel basically all right about ourselves on most days. Unfortunately, the enormous emphasis in today's world on measured achievement prohibits many people, let alone ADHD / ADD adopted / looked after children, from enhancing some of their very innate and exceptional qualities. Having a wide variety of interests is not something teachers often acknowledge in a student; enjoying people who are unconventional or different in some way is usually seen as being "odd" rather than being broad-minded; schools rarely praise humour; and a good sense of direction probably goes entirely unnoticed. Yet, these are the kinds of attributes that can contribute to a person's self-worth even when so much else seems to go awry for them.

ADHD / ADD adopted / looked after children are so used to being told what they do wrong and what they forgot to do or did not do that they have little chance to develop confidence in themselves. ADHD / ADD children hear all of the time how annoying and frustrating their behaviour is for others, and children in care quite naturally assume that they were "not good enough", which is why they feel they were abused or neglected, and "given away". A few exceptionally resilient people do seem to rise above the pervasive negativity that comes their way, but most children determine their own sense of self via the mirror of how they see those around them seeing them. If we are consistently told that we are naughty or evil or that we are a "bad seed", there is really little reason not to believe that. For ADHD / ADD adopted / looked after children, this is a poor self-image that is contrived out of a faulty reflection rather than out of the reality of who they really are and what they might become.

In most instances, our self-image is enhanced when we can take responsibility for ourselves and our actions. All children who have attention dysfunctions will benefit from learning more about ADHD so they can begin to understand some of their behaviours and impulses and so they can recognize when and how to acquire assistance for controlling these actions. As adopted / looked after children with ADHD/ADD begin to gain insight into their personal histories and to understand why it is that attending and focusing on tasks is so difficult for them, they have a better chance of managing the difficulties and enhancing the strengths in their lives.

Self-esteem does not arrive on our doorstep in a single package. Our concept of who we are is made up of many pieces that are highly fluid and constantly changing, and that derive out of experience over time. A poor self-image need not be all encompassing, and certainly is not irreversible. The process of change is slow, however, and it is a drop-by-drop metamorphosis. Sensitive parents/carers and supportive teachers/schools are vital links in this process, but, ultimately, it might actually be a friend who will help make the most difference in the young life of an adopted/looked after child with ADHD/ADD.

At the end of the day, we cannot ever really make a friend for our child, but there are some things that we can teach them that might enable them to improve their relationship-making skills. It is also quite important to recognize that many healthy, happy people with good self-images choose not to have large groups of friends. They are content with one or two good friends, and that works for them. The difference is that they choose to have two rather than ten friends, while ADHD/ADD adopted/looked after children do not know how to make one, two, or ten friends. Once we help them learn how to be a friend and have a friend, they will be in a position to choose how many people they enjoy having around them.

Being and becoming a friend

Ask children why so-and-so is their friend, and they almost always say something to the effect of, "She's nice." Depending upon the age and maturity of the child, more qualities will be added and described, so that a child might say:

- she listens to me;
- he's funny and makes me laugh;
- he understands me;
- she's always there for me;
- we like to do stuff together;
- we have a lot of the same interests.

Empathy and involvement in activities emerge from this list as important factors in friendships. Therefore, those are among the qualities we need to teach. Since ADHD/ADD adopted/looked after children often lack empathy, it is good to think how such a complex concept and feeling might be communicated to a child. Once again, a certain neutrality works best in the beginning, and once more, too, books are often good entries into the feelings of others. For small children, animal characters are very often used representatively, as it is much easier for a child to look at a difficult issue or emotion outside of him/herself. Mercer Mayer's, *I Was So Mad!* (1983) is a good example of how one can look at feelings with a child through a storybook, but this is only one small example and there are many, many books which can be helpful. Films are good for older children and books on tape can be instructive when trying to listen to the tone of voice a character uses when upset or excited or pleased.

Keeping calm

Children who have trouble controlling their emotions and impulsivity often benefit from various "calming techniques". For children who have a tendency to become over-stimulated, aggravated, anxious, and hyperactive, it is important for them to be able to calm themselves down enough to be able to interact with others in a quieter, easier manner. Knowing how to calm yourself can be a very helpful tool to have in your kit.

Sometimes massage is valuable for infants, while teens might do well in Yoga or Tai Chi classes. Various scents of oils or candles burning can be relaxing if the scent is either new to the child or reminiscent of something nice, rather than evoking an old and frightening memory. It was mentioned in the previous chapter that weight-bearing activities usually work positively for ADHD/ADD children in terms of helping their nervous systems to become better organized.

The following are some very general calming techniques that may be worth considering:

Having a quiet, but not necessarily isolated, space that the child can go to with a special blanket or soft toy or book.

Deep pressure:

Let the child roll him/herself up in a blanket like a hot dog. If the child will allow it, it is beneficial for the adult to be able to apply additional pressure to the rolled-up child, but if this is at all scary, it is not a good idea.

The child can put hands on head or shoulders and press down hard.

Bear hugs have a calming effect if the child perceives that as a happy and comfortable hug to receive.

Weight bearing:

Any activity that involves taking a lot of weight on limbs: chin-ups, wheelbarrow races, push-ups, arm wrestling while lying on one's tummy.

Taking a walk with a heavy backpack, or even sitting in class with a heavy backpack (because weighted vests can provide more constant sensory information).

Almost all of these "exercises" are ones that the child can do himself. For example, if Toby is feeling agitated while listening to a group of children talking about and planning an activity, he could simply pick up a few books and hold them in his arms, or he could stand and listen while putting his hands on his head and applying pressure to the top of his head. Both of these small actions will help him to feel just that little bit steadier. When children are calmer and when they receive more accurate sensory information, they are in a better emotional and physical state to listen to and hear the feelings of others.

Hobbies, talents, skills

Even if your child does not have a particular or outstanding talent such as playing an instrument or being an athletic star or acting superbly on the stage, it is worth considering helping the child to develop a hobby or interest that might appeal not only to your child, but also to other children. Collecting vinyl records from the 1950s seems to be an "in thing" to do at the moment. Saving tickets from sports events, making funky jewellery, starting a new fad such as wearing different coloured socks on each foot, having an unusual pet, learning to juggle, or having a collection of bottle caps are all the kinds of hobbies and skills that children can quite readily develop or engage in. Some children have learned magic tricks; others have taught themselves how to plait hair in a special way; a child who liked to eat ice cream learned how to make ice cream.

Adrienne was fascinated by the wedding cake her foster mother made for a sister's wedding, so she decided she was going to learn how to decorate cakes. Adrienne's foster mother took advantage of this interest by inviting the next-door-neighbour girl over to their house, and she began teaching the two girls how to make decorations with icing. Soon, another girl heard about this, and eventually it became a small group event, providing Adrienne with a social life she had never had before, and vastly increasing her self-esteem.

The possibilities for helping children to develop interests and hobbies are endless, but they require creative thinking and endurance, because a lot of them will not actually work. Either the ADHD / ADD adopted / looked after child will give up or lose interest, or the "friend" no longer wants to continue, or the activity runs its own course. No reason to stop there, though! Just keep trying because each of you will discover many new projects and ideas in the process. Maybe one or more of these efforts will attract at least a temporary friend for your child, and many of them will boost the child's self esteem because she will realize that she can learn something new and do it well. If the child does find something that seems to spark an interest for a bit, it is good for the parent to tell the teacher, so that the teacher will have an opportunity to expand the activity in the classroom and perhaps include a few more children in the ADHD / ADD adopted / looked after child's circle of friends.

Considerable research has concluded that leisure activities can help to contribute to children's educational success, which is vitally important, but there is also some indication that finding outside school interests can help to link children socially with other young people who share these interests and activities, and who potentially can become friends. A relaxed atmosphere in which a child can enjoy the company of others in a common pursuit has the potential to enhance the child's self-confidence and social skills. These are accomplishments that will stay with them throughout their lives.

As with everything else discussed throughout this book, there are no easy answers and no guarantees. The ability to relate to at least one other human being is a strong desire for most people. For some, this is not a difficult task; for others it is a monumental challenge. The ADHD/ADD adopted/looked after child more often than not comes on to the social scene with a rather hefty handicap, so everything that adults who care for them, teach them, and work with them can do to get them off the driving range and on to the putting green will surely benefit their social score.

CHAPTER SIX

Conclusions

The power of the past

As a teenager, Christie began to come to terms with the fact that her childhood may not have been ideal, but that it was over. She also started to appreciate that both she and Daniel have attention deficits, probably genetically, and certainly aggravated by their chaotic and abusive early lives. Although never adopted, after several moves, Christie is living in long-term foster care very satisfactorily. She has worked for years with a therapist who has been able to help her close some of the chapters of her former life. While she does not throw away the key to those chapters, they are, nevertheless, put away and locked up, enabling her to move forward more successfully. She eventually connected with a caring occupational therapist who mentors her as well as helping her with her sensory integration difficulties. School was not Christie's greatest achievement, but she did stay through GCSEs and subsequently has been able to go to college, learning to become a book-keeper, as her facility with numbers stayed with her throughout her school years.

Although Christie elected not to have Contact with her mother, she and Daniel finally have been able to see one another on a regular basis. With the help of the therapist, they have established a very sound and congenial relationship. Christie continues to be uncomfortable socially, having made several false starts with friendships, but never having had the confidence to really share and relate to her peers. She still is a "loner," but feels that might change in time as she now has more self-confidence from having made so many other positive steps forward in her life.

Christie finds that having an attention deficit gets in her way in almost every aspect of her life other than her work with numbers, which is the only time she manages to concentrate diligently and happily. She is learning to use diaries and technological aids that facilitate her being able to get to college and appointments on time. Her foster carers have been supportive and innovative throughout all of Christie's difficulties, her periods of withdrawal, her leaps forward and her steps out of insecurity into a brighter future.

Finding a future

With great endurance on everyone's part, Daniel's adoption has not disrupted. He has been helped to stay in secondary school by his adoptive parents' extraordinary endeavours to get him extra help and outside tutoring, as well as periodic family therapy. In addition, they have channelled Daniel's aggressive energy by having him in a boxing club, run by their neighbour, who also grew up in the care system. The boxing coach has supported Daniel's efforts to make some friends, and Daniel's athletic talent has enabled other boys to admire him and look up to him.

Daniel does not want to accept the fact that he has ADHD, and insists that he is "just fine". Mostly, he continues to blame others for things that go wrong, and he is still often disruptive at school or in groups. He has had two teachers at school who were outstanding, and are probably the reason he has not dropped out, but his academic achievement is quite poor, and his social skills are marginal.

On the bright side, adoption is not something that Daniel denies. He has become very attached to Shirley and Marcus and is glad to have been adopted, although he misses his mother, whom he rarely sees. He agrees with Christie that she had a harder time in their birth home than he did, and feels guilty that she paid the price for him. Daniel does remember a lot of early beatings and frightening situations, but is comfortable now with Shirley and Marcus and behaves better when he is with them than when they are not around.

Daniel's parents worry about his future—when they have the time or energy to even think about it. While ADHD support groups and a connection with an adoptive parents' community have indeed been supportive and helpful, no one can answer the persistent question of whether or not, and how, Daniel will be able to live independently, and settle into a life that is viable and happy for him.

In essence, I have already written the "Conclusion" of this book into its Preface and reiterated it in each subsequent chapter. I began and I conclude with the premise that ADHD/ADD adopted/looked after children are potentially at risk, vulnerable youngsters, and, as such, we all need to think very carefully about them. On the one hand, the tendency might be to over-generalize our knowledge about them, forgetting that each of their experiences is so unique and often extraordinary that we must always remember to look at what each individual child's portrait is showing us. On the other hand, it is important not to ignore the important generalizations we do know that are applicable to the neurobiology and social–emotional development of children who suffer from attention problems and who have begun life in very compromised situations. As with Christie, the childhood of these children is past, and sometimes lost, but it is never over (Hayden, 1981).

While that is true for all of us, fortuitously, most of us do not walk into each new day with quite such heavy footsteps. For the ADHD/ADD adopted/looked after child, the suitcase of the past, bulging with hurtful memories and scary experiences, has a tendency to pop open unexpectedly and distastefully whenever something pulls on its catches. We all carry our childhood with us, and, for most of us, there are bits and pieces we would just as soon leave behind, but there are also many memories and stories that we are happy to use and to include as a foundation as we design our adult lives. We incorporate what we have learned from our parents and relatives and schools and communities into the bridges we construct as we build our adolescent and adult years. Children from troubled and compromised backgrounds do not have this luxury. Rather than sifting out just a few shattered bricks to throw away, they spend an enormous amount of energy and time trying to find even one remnant from their early years that they can happily hold on to. More extremely than for most of us, the ADHD/ADD adopted/looked after child and his/her family will find that growing up healthily and happily is a very slow walk through the forest which requires considerable path-retracing and few long steps forward. Progress and change are definitely possible, but not without plenty of stops for a rest or retreat, and with substantial scaffolding, along the way.

As a brief summary, it is helpful to remember that:

- adopted/looked after children with attention difficulties can be very complex and paradoxical youngsters;
- there are no easy answers when trying to understand them, helping to support them, or wanting to manage their behaviour with them;
- the more parents, carers, teachers, and other professionals can adjust the environment to respond to the needs of the individual child, the less conflict and the more chance for improvement there is likely to be;
- the brain is malleable and generous. Given optimal input, it will continuously make every effort to reorganize itself; but past experience lingers long. Many repetitions of new material are required;
- there is every reason to hope for a future that is an improvement over the past if the ingredients of change are consistent, kind, reliable, and trustworthy;
- friendships often remain problematic for these children and adults, with many of them going through life, not necessarily all alone, but not usually with the bevy of friends around them that they envy others for having.

This book has been focused primarily on the adoptive parents/carers and teachers of ADHD/ADD adopted/looked after children, because it is with these people that a child spends most of his/her time for the first sixteen or more years of life. On the other hand, for many in this group of children, there are also social workers, therapists, activity leaders, and community members who interact on a fairly consistent basis as well. I am particularly hopeful that the strategies and suggestions already presented will be incorporated into the therapeutic thinking of psychologists and psychiatrists who are involved with these children and their families. I also hope that many, or even a few, of the ideas will be useful to the wider community whose lives or work may be tangential to the ADHD/ADD adopted/looked after child and family.

As we have seen, the statistics of both ADHD/ADD children and of adopted/looked after children can be dismal. One hears, rightfully, that they are more prone to a large variety of antisocial behaviours and school failures; that they are disproportionately represented both in prison and on the street/homeless. They rank high among substance abusers, as teenage parents, and in the numbers of the unemployed. While these statistics are both undeniable and extremely costly to society, they are particularly unfortunate because, to a large extent, they are preventable. Countless dedicated parents, foster carers, teachers, therapists, and others have proved that the lives of ADHD/ADD adopted/looked after children can be improved through sensitive programmes of intervention. In the concept of "It takes a village to raise a child", friends and extended family and other members of the family's circle of contacts can make a bigger difference than they ever give credence to. It takes many helping hands to affect the lives of a traumatized child with attention difficulties, but it can be and has been done.

In order to engage families of complicated adopted/looked after children in therapeutic intervention, it is critical that therapists and teachers divest themselves of their inclination to work with parents as though it is the parents' "fault" that the ADHD/ADD adopted/looked after child behaves the way he/she does. In fact, very healthy relationships and families can be devastated by the enormity of the problems adopted and looked after children can bring with them, especially when they have attention disorders as well. It can be wonderfully helpful for adoptive parents and carers when they feel understood by others on the therapeutic team. Quinton, Rushton, Dance, and Mayes (1998) remind us that intervention that is not sufficiently intense might not have a strong enough impact to alter the outcome for the child (or the family). Similarly, conflict among those providing advice to parents and carers can be detrimental, whereas a cohesive and parent/carer involved approach has a much better chance of facilitating improvement for all concerned.

In the same vein that it would be useful and commendable to be able to prevent child abuse and neglect, Joel Nigg (2006), has succinctly asserted that: "Society has a huge stake in preventing ADHD and the worst outcomes that are associated with it" (p. 333).

The price to be paid for ignoring what we already know about how to prevent ADHD/ADD (exposure to lead, substance abuse, teratogenic influences in the environment, for example), and how to provide positive early interventions with unstable pregnant women is astronomical compared to the much lower cost of providing health, mental health and educational programmes that could prevent the elevated risks of psycho-social, emotional, academic, and behavioural dysfunction that we face today (Selwyn, Sturgess, Quinton, & Baxter, 2006). Perhaps not so coincidentally, many of the programmes that could help to prevent ADHD would also contribute to the prevention of child abuse and neglect.

Properly thought out and individualized early intervention programmes and therapies have been shown to make significant differences in the outcomes for children suffering from traumatic backgrounds and from attention disorders (Dozier & Manni, 2002). It is primarily the "untreated" children—those who do not receive appropriate interventions—who make up the staggering and frightening statistics of seriously problematic behaviour and of mental health dysfunction. Prevention is critical, and co-operative, knowledgeable intervention is mandatory.

Even though the focus of this book has not been on either diagnosis or prevention, it is obvious that these are both enormously important topics to debate and discuss. The intention of the book, however, has been about intervention and how any or all of us can provide interventions that really do make a difference. Importantly, we must believe that it is never too late to intervene, and that it is always worth making the effort to do so. Even though we cannot erase the errors of the past, we can certainly create a brighter future. Every child deserves the opportunity to decrease the elevated risks that a traumatized early childhood and attention disorders, whether neurologically and/or environmentally influenced, can create.

As we have seen, ADHD/ADD adopted/looked after children continuously respond to the environment that they have experienced and that they perceive. In order to rewire their neural pathways and to create a new mapping system, the child's physical and emotional environments must be altered. It is only in this manner that the brain will have a means of reorganizing the interpretation of messages that are sent its way. Therefore, it is not just the parents'/carers' responsibility at home, and not even just the school's job and the therapists' interventions that can cumulatively make a difference in each child's life. The role of extended family, friends and neighbours cannot be under-estimated either, as it is so often one or more of these people who can play a critical, sometimes even life-changing, part in a child's life. Supporting the parents, carers, and siblings of children in need of special or additional attention is also one small way of helping both the child and the family.

In addition to, or in lieu of, doing something specific with the ADHD/ADD adopted/looked after child, it can be extremely helpful if a friend or neighbour spends time with one or more of the siblings in the family. Sometimes, just taking a sibling for an outing, or giving that child private time, can be a powerful adjunct to making things better at home. Inviting the family to dinner, or babysitting, or including the family in a party or neighbourhood get-together is a larger gift than one might imagine. The strength of a community can prove extremely supportive and bonding. Families with special needs children will be exceptionally grateful to those who notice them and help them, even if it is only once in a while.

In a better world, parents and carers of children with ADHD/ADD and of children who are in or have been in the care system will be able to receive training specific to ADHD/ADD and to issues of early childhood development, including attachment, separation, the impact of neurological impairments, and sensitive behaviour management. They will also have access to individual and family counselling from therapists who are trained in the field of attention disorders and who have experience in working with children in care/children who are adopted. In what should not be a utopian world, children must be able to have thorough medical and psycho-educational investigations that can contribute to an understanding of how they are functioning and that can offer appropriate intervention guidelines, addressing the needs of the individual child both at home and at school.

* * *

In conclusion, I would like to share the following personal experience. For the past ten years, I have owned and directed a centre for families who foster and adopt. The Centre is called Our Place because that is what I believe it should be—a place where families and professionals can come together as equal contributors to the support and success of the children and parents/carers who share our family and theirs together. It is to these families I have dedicated *Searching to Be Found*, and it is with one of their stories that I would like to conclude.

* * *

When the bell rang, I was surprised to see Betsy Tesno at the door because she usually phones before coming in. Oliver was wrapped around her legs like Velcro, and both looked sad and forlorn.

"I slapped him," Betsy blurted out the moment I shut the door behind her, and then she burst into uncontrollable sobs. "How could I do that to him?"

Oliver stayed glued to his adoptive mother and didn't say a word. Sorrow was written all over him.

We all went upstairs to the sitting room, and I asked them to wait a moment while I went to collect a few toys for Oliver. He is six years old, incredibly clever, a hard piece of work. Oliver is one of those children many teachers neither like nor understand because he is perpetually naughty at school, extremely bright, and has few friends.

Ever since I had known this family, sleep—or the lack of it—has been problematic. Oliver's very chaotic and abusive background contributed to his fear of sleep, while his attention deficit slotted him into the category of ADHD children who "don't sleep". Again, like many ADHD boys, Oliver was unable to amuse himself safely when awake. He was a child who loved to take things apart, but there seemed to be nothing out of his range with regard to what would intrigue him. Electrical sockets were fair game, along with radios, tape recorders, clocks, or kitchen appliances. Each time Oliver woke up and got up at night, it naturally disturbed his younger brother, Dominic, as well, and inevitably it resulted in Betsy being up or on high alert the better part of every night.

When Betsy and Jack first adopted Oliver, they came frequently to Our Place and became a family we knew well. Although they adored Oliver from the time they first met him in the foster home when he was eighteen months old, they knew from the beginning that he was a lively and spirited child. Oliver came into the care system following an emergency hospitalization when his birth mother could no longer deal with his screaming, and had tried to suffocate him with a face flannel one afternoon when her partner was sleeping. Oliver's life was saved through the chance circumstance of a neighbour walking in to borrow milk at the very moment that Oliver's mother was stuffing the flannel into his mouth. He was nine months old at the time.

Oliver spent three days alone in hospital and was then moved to a foster home for a week while a more permanent placement was organized for him. He lived for the next nine months with very caring and competent foster carers who helped Betsy and Jack with Oliver's transition into their home. Two years later, Betsy and Jack took Dominic, then six months old, into their home from these same foster carers. Within the next year, they had legally adopted both boys, at which time Jack left home and moved out of the country with another woman. Betsy has been on her own with both boys since then.

Understandably, Betsy was often fraught and vastly overstretched. She was, and is, the most caring of mothers, and an extraordinarily kind and generous person. Although she has friends, most find Oliver too hard to manage, as does the school, so there is little reprieve for Betsy other than when she brings Oliver to Our Place for activities. Betsy has made several friends herself by coming to the Centre, and derives considerable support from the staff and from other mothers. Prior to this crisis, she and I had often discussed behaviour management. In addition, Oliver has regular consultations with the paediatrician, who monitors trials of medications, none of which has had long-term success, although some have improved Oliver's home and school behaviours for short periods of time.

* * *

With coffee, juice, biscuits, and toys in hand, I went back upstairs and sat down with Betsy and Oliver. When Oliver settled with a set of tools I'd brought him and when Betsy could catch her breath, this is the story she told.

Hearing a strange noise about two o'clock in the morning, Betsy cautiously got out of bed, for what amounted to the third time already that night, and found Oliver in the bathroom, where he was filling the tub and holding their cat under the water. As one can do in this kind of anger, exhaustion, and frustration, Betsy grabbed Oliver by the arm to get him away from the tub and the cat, and, in removing him, she wittingly, but uncontrollably, slapped him across the face with her other hand. At that point, he screamed, Dominic woke and began screaming as well, the cat jumped out of the tub and scratched Betsy, and water flew all over the bathroom. Betsy panicked upon realizing what she had done, and all three of them spent the rest of the night/morning in a state of shock.

Betsy knew she needed help, but did not know where to turn, being all too aware that what she had done was "reportable behaviour" to social services, and could result in removal of her children.

* * *

I use this family's story because it is poignantly representative of the state that adoptive parents/carers can find themselves in when children whose backgrounds and attention disorders are so complex and overwhelming, both to the child and to the family, that children incite behaviours in parents that parents would never dream possible of themselves. I do not believe in smacking children and neither does Betsy, but her having slapped Oliver was actually the least of my concerns when Betsy presented this incident to me.

One can only think of Oliver, who had been nearly suffocated himself, and who was drowning his cat at 2.30 in the morning; of Dominic, who was frightened by the drama of his mother's desperate tears and panic; of Betsy, who committed, in her eyes, the ultimate "crime" of "abusing" an abused child; and again, of Oliver, whose absence of internal control led to such violent and shocking behaviour that he scared himself as well as everyone else, and provoked a response from his mother that reignited his own sense of worthlessness and fear of losing the one person upon whom he had become so dependent and trusting.

* * *

Over the next year, I and others at Our Place worked quite intensely with this family, not specifically in "therapy sessions", but rather in a more holistic and global approach. Again, I use this family's story to describe and display the importance of a multi-modal intervention that extends to the school, community, and larger family in order to effect positive changes.

Oliver began to come weekly to our after school club—a small group of children who meet for one and a half hours once a week to do art, music, and cookery projects, and to learn to play together. The emphasis is on social (and a few basic academic) skills incorporated into playful, fun activities. The group is led on alternate weeks by a play therapist and a teacher of special needs children. While Oliver was involved in this group, Dominic had supervised play sessions with several other siblings of group members. Their sessions were led by a nursery nurse. Concomitantly, Betsy joined parents and carers who chatted together in our coffee room, forming a "natural" support group of very empathic men and women (mostly, but not exclusively, women).

During the next few months, I visited Oliver's school several times, had a couple of conferences with his teacher, and wrote numerous letters and reports in an effort to acquire additional help for Oliver and his teacher in the classroom. I also consulted frequently with the paediatrician, and Betsy periodically came in for an hour session individually with me. When this was not possible for her, either she phoned me or I rang her, just to check on her.

A teenager, who is adopted and had been coming to Our Place since she was a little girl, was now helping periodically in various activities. She became available for some part-time baby-sitting, which enabled Betsy to go out once in a while during the day just with Dominic. Sometimes she could leave Dominic with a neighbour, and was then able to meet up with her own friends for coffee. In the course of the year, Betsy's mother became ill, but a cousin who came to town to help her also became an important support person for Betsy.

Although it has not happened as yet, I am hopeful that Oliver will soon receive individual play therapy sessions on a regular basis. Clearly, this is a little boy who still has a lot to work out, but the intense input that has been provided for, and been well taken advantage of by, this family has made a substantial difference in their individual and overall functioning.

Importantly, it highlights the value of intervention. An adoption that could have disrupted, a child who was programmed for school failure, a family that was falling apart, have been given a very feasible chance to get back on track and to start in a new and healthier direction.

> *Betsy*: "The safety of coming to Our Place and the support of other mothers has sustained me."
>
> *Oliver*: "Please don't ever close Our Place. I want it to be here forever."
>
> *Dominic*: "I love to play here."
>
> *Oliver's teacher*: "You've made a huge difference in my understanding of Oliver. I'm really beginning to enjoy who he is."
>
> *Betsy's cousin*: "I really like the way the whole family can come to Our Place so that we can do things together and meet other families in the same situations."

The silence of their voices can only be heard by those who listen. As part of their village, we as professionals, families, friends, and citizens must be sure that we are hearing.

APPENDIX I

Characteristics of Attention Deficit (Hyperactivity) Disorder

Criteria extracted primarily from the *DSM-IV* (which differs slightly from the *DSM-IV-TR* 2000), with updated modifications from Russell Barkley's *Attention-deficit Hyperactivity Disorder: A Handbook for Diagnosis and Treatment* (3rd edn) 2005. New York: Guilford Press.

In order to receive a diagnosis of ADHD/ADD a child must exhibit at least six to eight of the following characteristics for a duration of a minimum of six months, and prior to the age of seven years. Although the criteria tend to vary somewhat, according to the researcher and author, and depending upon the country in which one is diagnosed, nevertheless, all concur that the symptoms of inattention must have persisted to a degree that is maladaptive and inconsistent with the child's developmental level. Moreover, the symptoms must manifest themselves pervasively across settings, causing impairments in major domains of life functioning—home, school, work. Difficulty with behaviour inhibition is considered central to the diagnosis of the disorder.

- Often fails to give close attention to details or makes careless mistakes in schoolwork, work, or other activities.

- Often has difficulty sustaining attention in tasks or play activities.
- Often does not seem to listen to what is being said to him/her.
- Often does not follow through on instructions and fails to finish schoolwork, chores, or duties in the workplace (not due to oppositional behaviour or failure to understand instructions).
- Often has difficulty organizing tasks and activities.
- Often avoids or expresses reluctance about or has difficulties in engaging in tasks that require sustained mental effort.
- Often loses things necessary for tasks or activities.
- Is easily distracted by extraneous stimuli.
- Often forgetful in daily activities.

The symptoms of hyperactivity–impulsivity must have persisted to a degree that is maladaptive and inconsistent with the child's developmental level.

Hyperactivity

- Often fidgets with hands or feet or squirms in seat.
- Leaves seat in classroom or in other situations in which remaining in seat is expected.
- Often runs about or climbs excessively in situations where it is inappropriate.
- Often has difficulty playing or engaging in leisure activities quietly.
- Is always on the go and acts driven.
- Often talks excessively.

Impulsivity

- Often blurts out answers to questions before they have been completed.
- Often has difficulty waiting in lines or waiting turns in games or group situations.
- Often interrupts or intrudes on others' games or conversations.

APPENDIX II

ADHD/ADD adults who are adopted or who grew up in care

Throughout this book, I have emphasized that many ADHD/ADD adopted/looked after children do well as adults, but I have also alluded to the fact that most of them still need some sort of adjunct help such as secretaries, partners, technology, and so forth. Below are some examples of why they do.

> Kevin, aged thirty-three, and Brian, aged thirty-six, have left for their summer holiday at a beach resort. Upon arriving, they discover that neither has brought a brush or comb. Kevin remembered to bring sandals, but no shorts; Brian has shorts, but neither sandals nor swimming trunks. Brian has "lost" his toothbrush and toothpaste between home and the resort.
>
> At the end of his four-day visit with a cousin who lives across the country, Larry, aged twenty-nine, is about to get out of the car at the airport when he discovers that he does not have his flight information with him. He knows the airline, but neither the time it leaves nor the flight number.
>
> Georgia, aged thirty-seven, is due to go to a formal dinner directly from work. Half hour before the end of the work day, her secretary mentions that she hasn't seen Georgia's dress for the evening and asks where it

is. Georgia, who lives forty-five minutes away from work—and from the location of the dinner—remembers that she has left the dress and all accessories on her bed at home.

After a productive tennis lesson, Alison, aged forty-one, decides that she will get up early the following morning to have a practice session before taking the children to school. Alison forgets to change her alarm clock, but when she wakes up at the usual hour, she realizes that she has left her tennis kit at her friend's house, and then one of her boys comes in to say she is late because he needed to be taken to school half hour earlier than usual that day.

Michael, aged thirty-five, spends the weekend going through a box of old school and camp paraphernalia. After long hours of reading through school reports and comments on papers, and after reviewing the camp counsellors' letters home to his parents, Michael says to his wife: "There is a lot that was said about me when I was young that is still pretty true about me." In answer to her questions about what was said, Michael responds: "Things like needing to be more organized and needing to stop wandering around the room and not talking to other kids during class. Stuff like paying more attention to what I'm doing and getting things done on time."

Steve's father comments that it is still a lot of work to have Steve, aged forty-three, come for a holiday at their house. "He is well intentioned," says Steve's dad, "but he just never does what he says he is going to do—activities he himself would like to do! He doesn't really know how to help around the house, so we still have to ask him or remind him to do basic things that anyone else his age would do automatically. We also have to wait for him for every single thing we do with him."

Grace says that her work itself is not a problem for her because she is a fashion designer, something she has loved doing from the time she was little. On the other hand, at thirty-eight years of age, she feels discouraged that everything around the job continues to be so difficult: remembering appointments, getting jobs done on time, being where she is supposed to be when she is told to be there, getting directions and specifications down exactly. Grace frequently loses jobs, but her design is consistently admired.

Randall relays that he makes very poor judgements about people and situations. He feels that he is not good at "reading" people well, and he is beginning to realize how gullible he can be. Moreover, despite his thirty-two years, Randall has been unable to manage a bank account or a credit card, so keeps cash at home and pays only in cash. This is not his preference, but he just cannot organize himself well enough to keep a bank account solvent.

These are only a few of the many situations that one hears about when listening to adults who continue to find their ADHD/ADD problematic. Adoption issues come into play much more subtly, and except for those who say they have to watch their temper, the stories from adopted adults, or adults who grew up in care and who now are leading functional lives, are not so frequently described in explicit adoption/looked after terms as are ADHD/ADD stories. For many, issues arise when they have their own children, when they need to think about disciplining their children, when extended family issues come into play, when they feel bullied at work; but none of these stories are relayed quite so specifically as are their examples of how ADHD/ADD gets in the way of their lives.

For the most part, the vignettes above are told by adults who, indeed, are struggling with various issues, but who are also managing to work and to socialize in quite acceptable ways—some much more so than others, of course.

APPENDIX III

Helpful suggestions for teachers and parents/carers

The following suggestions represent an amalgamation of the kinds of lists one usually sees pertaining to the ways in which parents, carers, and teachers can help ADHD / ADD adopted / looked after children.

- Be aware not to over-stimulate or over-exhaust.
- Limit possibilities of distraction and diversion, but keep things moving and engaging.
- Prioritize one or two target behaviours for immediate management.
- Contain negative behaviours rather than attempting to eliminate them all at one time.
- Be consistent and predictable about rules and routines, causes and consequences.
- Reward what is specifically well done—use positive reinforcement frequently.
- Provide structure and planned programmes that help children to organize and monitor their own behaviours.
- Establish schedules that build in frequent and physically active breaks.

- Offer choice, and allow for flexibility within the structure.
- Prepare the child for "what happens next".
- Have a personal code system between the teacher and the child or the parent and the child for monitoring in-class or other social behaviours.
- Play games and do exercises that practise desired behaviours.
- Write directions down as well as giving them orally. Ask the child to repeat the instructions.
- Use pictures and manipulatives in teaching and explaining.
- Understand and tolerate mistakes. Use them for learning.
- Support and teach study techniques, organizational habits, and problem-solving strategies.
- Allow a child to change work sites frequently.
- Help child to formulate a plan before undertaking a task and to evaluate the plan after its completion.
- Avoid statements like: "You could do this if you tried harder."
- Permit the child to do something with his/her hands while engaging in a long period of listening.
- Provide many opportunities for child to create, use imaginative thinking, and to receive recognition for originality.
- Intervene and support the child so that he/she is prevented from becoming humiliated at school or in the neighbourhood.
- Recognize that change can represent something especially big, often negative, sometimes scary to these children. Neither adopted/looked after nor ADHD/ADD children make transitions easily.
- Teachers: family trees, Mother's Day cards, autobiographies, grandparent interviews, baby pictures, time-lines, and early memory stories do not have to be eliminated, but they do need re-evaluating.

APPENDIX IV

Resources

The books and resources listed below are all independent of those in the References of this book as the references include only sources that were cited in the text. Above and beyond those books and articles, there is much of value to read. A difficulty with listing additional materials is that one will inevitably leave out particular resources that are equally as important and useful as those which have been included—or which some readers may feel are even more valuable than the citations I have selected. I apologize for this, and emphasize that the following lists are made up of authors, organizations, and other reading materials that have been particularly important to me as I have searched, read, learnt, and talked about attention disorders and about adoption and fostering.

Professional Reading

Barkley, R. All or any of his work on ADHD/ADD.
Cattanach, A. (1992). *Play Therapy with Abused Children*. London: Jessica Kingsley.
Fahlberg, V. All or any of her work on adoption issues.

Gil, E. (1991). *The Healing Power of Play: Working with Abused Children.* New York: Guilford.

Gil, E. (2006). *Helping Abused and Traumatized Children.* New York: Guilford.

James, B. (1989). *Treating Traumatized Children.* New York: Free Press.

Kewley, G. (2001). *Attention Deficit Hyperactivity Disorder: Recognition, Reality & Resolution.* London: David Fulton.

Levine, M. All or any of his work on learning disorders / ADHD / ADD

McKinstry, L. (2005). A very different view of ADHD from England! *Pediatrics, 115*(5): 1272.

Melina, L. R. (2002). *Raising Adopted Children.* New York: HarperCollins.

Perry, B. All or any of his work on trauma and the brain. See website below.

Richards, A. (2003). *ADHD: A Challenging Journey.* London: Chapman Educational.

Schofield, G., Beek, M., Sargent, K., & Thoburn, J. (2000). *Growing Up in Foster Care.* London: BAAF.

Smith, C. (1983). *Learning Disabilities: The Interaction of Learner, Task and Setting.* New York: Little, Brown.

Stern, D. (1985). *The Interpersonal World of the Infant.* New York: Basic Books.

Gillian Schofield, David Howe, David Quinton, Julie Selwyn are all contemporary British researchers who have contributed enormously to the field of adoption / fostering. Professionals wanting to read the most current information in the field would do well to refer to any of these researchers.

Attention Deficit Hyperactivity Disorder Information Services (ADDISS), is Great Britain's largest support and resource group for those dealing with ADHD / ADD and is an excellent contact for both professionals and parents / carers wanting to know more about attention deficit disorders. www.addiss.co.uk

British Adoption and Fostering (BAAF) and Adoption UK are the national resources for both parents / carers and professionals concerned with adoption and fostering. www.baaf.org.uk and www.adoptionuk.org

The Evan B. Donaldson Institute, in the USA, provides leadership that improves adoption laws, policies and practices through research, education, and advocacy. www.adoptioninstitute.org

Parent/teacher reading

Auer, C., & Blumberg, S. (2006). *Parenting a Child with Sensory Processing Disorder.*San Francisco, CA: New Harbinger.

Cooper, P., & Ideus, K. (1997). *Attention Deficit Hyperactivity Disorder—A Practical Guide for Teachers.* London: Jessica Kingsley.

Du Paul, G., & Stoner, G. (1994). *ADHD in the Schools.* London: Guilford, School Practitioner Series.

Hayden, T. Any of her beautifully sensitive books depicting her work with severely traumatized children.

Hughes, L. (2007). *Understanding and Supporting Children with ADHD.* London: Chapman Educational.

Jones, C., Searight, H. R., & Urban, M. A. (1999). *Parent Articles about ADHD.* San Antonio, TX: Communication Skill Builders.

Levine, M. (2003). *The Myth of Laziness.* New York: Simon & Schuster.

Lougy, R., DeRuva, S., & Rosenthal, D. (2007). *Teaching Young Children with ADHD.* Thousand Oaks, CA: Corwin.

Winnicott, D. W. (1971). *Playing and Reality.* New York: Penguin.

Wood, L., & Ng, N. (Eds.) (2000). *Adoption and the Schools: Resources for Parents and Teachers.* Available from Families Adopting in Response, PO Box 51436, Palo Alto, California 94303.

Children

BRAKES—newsletter for Kids with ADHD. Edited by Patricia Quinn and Judith Stern. Washington, DC: Magination Press

Gavin, M. (1998). *Otto Learns about His Medicine: A Story about Medication for Hyperactive Children.* Washington, DC: Magination Press.

Gordon, M. (1992). *My Brother's a World Class Pain: A Sibling's Guide to ADHD/Hyperactivity.* New York: GSI Publications.

Gordon, M. (1995). *I'd Rather Be With A Real Mom Who Loves Me: A Story for Foster Children.* New York: GSI Publications. (Foster carers, be sure to read this book by yourself first and judge whether or not it is appropriate for your particular child.)

Hillyer, Ed. (2001). *Streaky:The Annoying Little Piglet.* London: Royal College of Psychiatrists.

Weaver, Chris. (1998). *Full of Beans.* Australia: Shrinkrap Publishers.

Videos/websites

Video: *Hyperactive Children in the Classroom*. 1999. 35 minutes. Margaret Thompson, Elaine Cronk. Emphasizes how isolated parents feel in the school and community.

Video: *Kids in the Corner*. 1999.Tiger Aspect Production.

(Both of the videos listed above are available through ADDISS.)

Video: FAT City, Richard Lavoie Public Television. USA.

www.adder.org.uk

www.addiss.co.uk

www.addwarehouse.com Good catalogue of games and learning resources.

www.casey.org Their mission is to improve foster care and to prevent the need for foster care. See their publication: *Improving Family Foster Care*.

www.chadd.org (CHADD = Children and Adults with Attention Deficit/Hyperactivity Disorder).

www.childrentherapytoys.com

www.childtrauma.org. Dr Bruce Perry.

www.fairfamilies.org

www.nice.org.uk have a section on ADHD.

www.oaasis.co.uk

www.odsacone.org There are many school related titles on this website.

www.sign.ac.uk (Scottish Intercollegiate Network) *Attention Deficit & Hyperkinetic Disorders in Children and Young People*. 2001.

www.spence-chapin.org They have an adoption resource centre.

REFERENCES

Adesman, A. (2006). Expert advice: ADHD and adoption. Spence-Chapin services to families and children: www.spence-chapin.org www. LHJ.com.

American Academy of Child and Adolescent Psychiatry: Facts for Families (2004). *Children who can't pay attention/ADHD*. www.aacap.org (accessed July).

Ayres, J. (1973). *Sensory Integration and Learning Disorders*. Los Angeles, CA: Western Psychological Services.

Barkley, R. (1996). Critical issues in research on attention. In: G. R. Lyon & N. Krasnegor (Eds.), *Attention, Memory and Executive Function*. Baltimore, MD: Paul H. Brookes.

Barkley, R. (2002). Psychosocial treatments for attention-deficit/hyperactivity disorder in children. *Journal of Clinical Psychiatry, 63*(Suppl. 12): 36–43.

Barkley, R. (2005) *Taking Charge of ADHD: The Complete Authoritative Guide for Parents* (3rd edn). New York: Guilford.

Becker-Weidman, A. (2007). Child abuse and neglect: effect on child development, brain development, and interpersonal relationships. www.adoptionarticlesdirectory.com, accessed 21 August.

Biederman, J., Faraone, S. V., Keenan, K., Benjamin, J., Krifcher, B., Moore, C., Sprich-Buckminster, S., Ugaglia, K., Jellinek, M. S., Steingard,R., et al. (1992). Further evidence for family-genetic risk factors in attention deficit hyperactivity disorder patterns of comorbidity in probands and relative psychiatrically and pediatrically referred samples. *Archives of General Psychiatry, 49*: 728–738.

Borkowski, M. (2006). *Understanding the Complexities of Contact for Adopted and Looked After Children*. Bristol: Our Place.

Brodzinsky, D. M., & Schechter, M. D. (Eds.) (1990). *The Psychology of Adoption*. Oxford: Oxford University Press.

Brookner, A. (1989). *Latecomers*. London: Grafton.

Brooks, R. (1991). *The Self-Esteem Teacher*. Circle Pines, MN: American Guidance Service.

Browning, G. (2006). *How to . . . Concentrate*. The *Guardian*, September.

Cairns, K. (2002). *Attachment, Trauma and Resilience: Therapeutic Caring for Children*. London: British Adoption and Fostering.

Cairns, K., & Stanway, C. (2004). *Learn the Child*. London: British Adoption and Fostering.

Carter, P. (2006). Behaviour problems in the looked after child. West Midlands British Association for Adoption and Fostering Conference, July 2006.

Comfort, R. (1992). *Teaching The Unconventional Child*. Denver, CO: Libraries Unlimited.

Comfort, R. (1997). When nature didn't nurture, what's a foster/adoptive family to do? *Infants and Young Children, 10*(2): 27–35.

Comfort, R. (2007). For the love of learning: promoting educational achievement for looked after and adopted children. *Adoption & Fostering, 31*(1): 28–34.

De Posada, J., & Singer, E. (2005). *Don't Eat the Marshmallow . . . Yet!* New York: Penguin.

Department for Education and Skills (DfES) (2006). *Meeting the Needs of Disabled Pupils*. London: DfES.

Department for Education and Skills (DfES) (2007). *Care Matters: Time for Change White Paper*. London: DfES.

Diagnostic and Statistical Manual of Mental Disorders, 4th Edition (2000). Washington, DC: American Psychiatric Association.

Diamond-Berry, K. (2007). The consequences of intergenerational chemical addiction on infants, toddlers and families. *Zero To Three Bulletin, 27*(4): 5–10.

Dozier, M., & Manni, M. (2002). Recognizing the special needs of infants' and toddlers' foster parents: development of a relational intervention. *Zero To Three Bulletin, 22*: 7–13.

Fahlberg, V. (1995). *A Child's Journey Through Placement*. London: British Adption and Fostering.

Faraone, S., & Doyle, A. (2001). The nature and heritability of attention-deficit-hyperactivity disorder. *Child Adolescent Psychiatry Clinic, 10*: 299–316.

Fugard, A. (1983). *Tsotsi*. London: Penguin.

Ge, X., Conger, R. D., Cadoret, R. J., Neiderhiser, J. M. (1996). The developmental interface between nature and nurture. A mutual influence model of child antisocial behavior and parent behaviors. *Developmental Psychology, 32*(4): 574–589.

Geddes, H. (2006). *Attachment in the Classroom: The Links between Children's Early Experience, Emotional Well Being and Performance in Schools*. London: Worth.

Glaser, D. (2000). Child abuse and neglect and the brain—a review. *Journal of Child Psychology and Psychiatry, 41*(1): 97–116.

Glennen, S., & Bright, B. (2005). Five years later: language in school-age internationally adopted children. *Seminars in Speech and Language, 26(*1): 86–101.

Golding, K. (2004). Children experiencing adverse parenting early in life. The story of attachment. *Clinical Psychology, 40*, 21–23.

Golding, K., Dent, H., Nissim, R., & Stott, L. (2006). *Thinking Psychologically about Children Who Are Looked After and Adopted*. Chichester: Wiley.

Grant, L. (2006). *The People on the Street*. London: Virago.

Gunnar, M. (2001). Effects of early deprivation: findings from orphanage-reared infants and children. In: C. A. Nelson & M. Luciana (Eds.), *Handbook of Developmental Cognitive Neuroscience* (pp. 617–629). Cambridge, MA: MIT Press.

Hayden, T. (1981). *Somebody Else's Kids*. New York: Avon Publishing.

Healy, J. (1990). *Endangered Minds*. London: Simon & Schuster.

Heineman, T. V. (1998). *The Abused Child*. New York: Guilford.

Hoban, R. (1969). *Best Friends for Frances*. New York: Harper Row.

Huang-Storms, L., David, R., Dunn, J., & Bodenhauer-Davis, E. (2005). Neuro feedback in the treatment of children with histories of relational trauma. *Journal of Neurotherapy, 9*(4): 125–127

Jackson, S. (Ed.) (2001). *Nobody Ever Told Us School Mattered: Raising the educational Attainments of Children in Care*. London: BAAF.

Jackson, S. (Ed). (2007). Special Issue: *Education, Adoption & Fostering, British Adoption and Fostering, 31*(1).

Jackson, S., & McParlin, P. (1998). Surviving the care system: education and resilience. *Journal of Adolescence, 21*: 561–583.

Jackson, S., & McParlin, P. (2006). The education of children in care. *The Psychologist, 19*(Spring): 90–93.

Johnson, D. E. (2000). Medical and developmental sequelae of early childhood institutionalisation in Eastern European countries. The effects of early adversity in neurobehavioral development. *The Minnesota Symposia on Child Psychology, 31*: 113–162.

Juffer, F., & van Ijzendoorn, M. H. (2005). Behavior problems and mental health referrals of international adoptees. *Journal of the American Medical Association, 293*: 2501–2515.

Kay, J. (1998). *The Trumpet*. London: Picador.

Kirby, D., & Honeywood, D. (2007). The entrepreneurial tendencies of young people with ADHD and traditional students: are those with ADHD nascent entrepreneurs? ADDISS Conference, London, May.

Lansdown, R., Burnell, A., & Allen, M. (2007). Is it that they won't do it, or is it that they can't? Executive functioning and children who have been fostered and adopted. London: *Adoption and Fostering, 31*(2): 44–52.

Lavoie, R. (2006). *It's So Much Work to Be Your Friend*. New York: Touchstone, Simon & Schuster.

Lehmann, C. (2002). Abuse said to interfere with child brain development. *Psychiatric News, 37(*1): 23.

Levine, M. D. (1987). *Developmental Variation and Learning Disorders*. Cambridge, MA: Educators Publishing Service.

Lloyd, G., Stead, J., & Cohen, D (Eds.) (2006). *Critical New Perspectives on ADHD*. London: Routledge.

Lobell, A. (1979). *Frog and Toad Are Friends*. New York: Harper & Row.

Look Before You Leap (children's game) (1994). New York: Childswork/Childsplay.

Lowry, C. (2007). New insights into the brain. *Research Review, April*.

Marshall, J. (1972). *George and Martha*. New York: Houghton Mifflin.

Mayer, M. (1983). *I Was So Mad!*. Wisconsin, IL: Golden Books.

McCaskill, C. (2002). *Safe Contact? Children in Permanent Placement and Contact with Their Birth Relative*. London: Russell House.

Minarik, E. H. (1958). *No Fighting, No Biting!* New York: Harper Trophy.

Mitchell, A. (1984). Back in the Playground Blues in *On the Beach at Cambridge*, Alison & Busby: London.

National Clearinghouse on Child Abuse and Neglect Information, National Adoption Information Clearinghouse (2001). Washington, DC: October.

Nigg, J. T. (2006). *What Causes ADHD?* New York: Guilford.

Perry, B. D., Runyan, D., & Sturges, C. (1998). Bonding and attachment in maltreated children: How abuse and neglect in childhood impact social and emotional development. *Caregiver Education Series, 1*(5): 1–12.

Perry, D. B. (2001). Violence and childhood: How persisting fear can alter the child's developing brain. In: D. Schetky & E. Benedek (Eds.), *Textbook of Child and Adolescent Forensic Psychiatry* (pp. 221–138). Washington, DC: American Psychiatric Press.

Quinton, D., Rushton, A., Dance, C., & Mayes, D. (1998). *Joining New Families: A Study of Adoption and Fostering in Middle Childhood.* Chichester: Wiley.

Rutter, M. (1998). Developmental catchup and deficit, following adoption after severe global early deprivation, *Journal of Child Psychology and Psychiatry, 39*: 465–476.

Selwyn, J., & Quinton, D. (2004). Stability, permanence, outcomes and support. *Adoption and Fostering, 28*(4): 6–15.

Selwyn, J., Sturgess, W., Quinton, D., & Baxter, C. (2006). *Costs and Outcomes of Non-infant Adoptions.* London: BAAF.

Shonkoff, J., & Phillips, D. (Eds). (2000). *From Neurons to Neighborhoods.* Washington, DC: National Academy Press.

Silver, J., Amster, B., & Haecker, T. (1999). *Young Children and Foster Care.* Baltimore, MD: Brookes.

Silver, L. (1999). The Misunderstood Child. New York: McGraw Hill.

Simmel, C., Brooks, D., Barth, R. P., & Hinshaw, S. P. (2001). Externalizing symptomatology among adoptive youth: prevalence and preadoption risk factors. *Journal of Abnormal Child Psychology, 29*(1): 57.

Smart, J. (2003). *Adoptive Parents' Guide to the Special Needs Child.* No. 13. Ontario: Hilborn

Smith, C. (2001). *Learning Disabilities A to Z.* New York: The Free Press.

Sprich, S., Biederman, J., Crawford, M. H., Mundy, E., & Faraone, S. (2000). Adoptive and biological families of children and adolescents with ADHD, *Journal of the American Academy of Child and Adolescent Psychiatry, 39*(11): 1432.

Stein, S. M., & Chowdhury, U. (2006). *Disorganized Children.* London: Jessica Kingsley.

Stock-Kranowitz, C. (2005). *The Out-of-Sync Child.* New York: Penguin.

Teicher, M. D. (2000). Wounds that time won't heal: The neurobiology of child abuse. *Cerebrum*: The Dana Forum on brain science. 2(4): 50–67.

The Who Cares? Trust (2003). *Education Matters—For Everyone Working with Children in the Looked After System*. London: The Who Cares? Trust.

Weaver, C. (Ed.) (1994). *Success at Last!* Portsmouth, NH: Heinemann.

Webster-Stratton, C. (1999). *How to Promote Children's Social and Emotional Competence.* London: Paul Chapman.

INDEX

For Product Safety Concerns and Information please contact our EU representative GPSR@taylorandfrancis.com
Taylor & Francis Verlag GmbH, Kaufingerstraße 24, 80331 München, Germany

www.ingramcontent.com/pod-product-compliance
Ingram Content Group UK Ltd.
Pitfield, Milton Keynes, MK11 3LW, UK
UKHW022202190926
475702UK00003B/163
* 9 7 8 0 3 6 7 3 2 6 7 4 6 *